'I only wanted to be a Dad'

© 2018 VASPX Steve Petrou.

Isbn: 978-0-9569076-5-3

To our little angels Xristos and Andrea. You are forever in our hearts.

To Petros, my beacon of hope.

To Vas, my beacon to a better me.

To my dad. God Bless you and may you rest in peace.

Authors:

VASPX: Vaspx is terror and hope; also, pain and faith. You will understand who Vaspx is, at the end of the book.

Contributing author: **Dr. Robin Hadley**

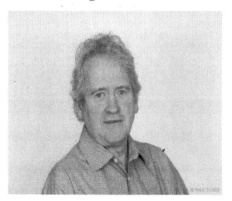

Robin was awarded his PhD in Social Gerontology by Keele University in December 2015. His PhD study into the experiences of involuntarily childless older men, has received much international media attention. Robin's previous careers included roles as counsellor, deputy technical manager, scientific and technical photographer, kitchen assistant, and bar tender. Robin's training as a counsellor and his own experience of the desire for fatherhood led him to research into the desire for fatherhood in involuntarily childless men as part of his Master of Arts in Counselling at The University of Manchester. He followed this up with a self-funded Master of Science (again at The University of Manchester) exploring the levels of desire for parenthood ('broodiness') in females and males, parents and non-parents. He is in demand as a research consultant and has recently completed projects relating to aging, dementia, technology, fathers, and childlessness. He was born in 1960's in a working class area of Manchester and enjoys football, cricket, theatre, and bird watching.

Special thanks to:

Chris Thorne – he was there from the beginning. He has finished university, started a full-time job, and handed his resignation to me four times. I shall never accept it!

Andreas Paphiti – a psychology major, he helped change the focus of the book to emotions.

Ken Korczack – my Minnesota friend, who likes cooking.

Dee Wilkins – senior editor of IMMPACT magazine.

Vic Waghorn – actor, deep thinker, and a gentle soul.

Table of Contents

Prologue

1. About Me and 'I only wanted to be a Dad'

2. How It Started For Us

3. Infertility

4. Two Choices When You Decide to Try to Get Pregnant

5. Living with Infertility

6. Secondary infertility

7. I Was the King!

8. Sex and Infertility

9. Firing Blanks

10. Dealing with IVF

11. IVF

12. Anger and Arguments

13. Birth

14. Hate

15. Faith

9

16. Miscarriage or Losing a Fetus

17. Death

18. My Shame

19. The Telephone and Why Answering It was Always Bad News

20. Men Suffer Too

21. Salvation

22. The Later Years

23. Childlessness and Men Who wanted to be Dads—Dr. Robin Hadley

24. I am my Father's Son

25. My Personal Opinion

Epilogue

PROLOGUE

"It was the noblest of dreams; it was utter terror."

My name is Steve. My wife's name is Vaso (Vas), and I am here to tell you a story.

I've never raised my voice at my wife apart from this one time.

"Look at me."

Vas refused to look at me.

"Damn it, look at me!"

She knew we were facing complete annihilation. She was in the middle of it, still clinging to religion and hope. All I saw around me was death. My anger was beyond safe limits. My hands were shaking.

She finally looked at me.

"Are you out of your bloody mind?" I said. "You will die!"

I grabbed her hand and squeezed it hard. I stared at her without blinking.

"Please!" Vas said.

"You will all die! All of you." I squeezed her hand even harder. I just could not believe what I was hearing. "Listen to me and listen well. There is no bloody way I am going to let you do this."

"Please, Steve. It is their only chance!"

"None of you will have a bloody chance of surviving if you delay this. Do you hear me? None of you!"

"Please …"

Continuing to glare at her, my grip grew even harder. She had to understand that this was no debate. She was completely white, as the blood transfusions could not keep up. Any delay would have meant certain death for all of them.

On Wednesday, we were ecstatic. On Friday, two lousy days later, they threw us into the cesspit of death again.

Vas never stopped to consider me. Had I agreed with her decision, I would have been the only one walking out of that hospital, a beaten and broken man with only regrets, hate, and anger as companions.

I've never imagined that those words would've ever been uttered by me. That was never part of the plan.

When I was young, I planned to get a lucrative job, a classy sports car, marry a great girl I was crazy about, buy a comfortable house and have a family. I spent much time contemplating and planning about the job, the car, and, of course, the girl. As far as having a family went, for a whole five seconds, I settled on maybe two children. That was the last part of the jigsaw and the easiest. Simple or so I thought.

What were your plans in adolescence or what are your plans now?

I got the car, set up my own business, bought the house, and married the girl. The hard part was done. Now I was all set for the enjoyable and fun time of having a baby.

How many times have you driven past a house and seen kids playing and laughing out the front or you glanced through a window and saw a family eating dinner or watching the television?

I witnessed this scene countless times. I expected that when I was older I would be part of it. Why would I not be? My parents, friends, and virtually everyone I knew had their family without problems.

Unknown to me, however, I was part of a little-known club. In America, it is called the One-in-Eight, and in some other countries, it is the One-in-Six. It is called the 'infertility club'.

Here is the kicker: All that planning and all those sacrifices in order to achieve my goals were for nought. The job, the car, and the house meant nothing if I could not have a baby.

My wife and I were at a party. Low, soft music played in the background, and there was food and drink provided on the surrounding tables. Infertility had been an unwelcome companion for a year now. I was talking to some friends.

Frank, "My new car is awesome. You'll not believe the extras it's got." Every couple of years, Frank gets a new car and goes to great lengths to show off.

George, "Does it drive itself like the car in the Knight Rider?"

Everyone smiles apart from Frank.

George, "I split up with Mary. I am with Marlene now who's a redhead. " George is the only one of our friends who is unmarried.

Every time we meet, he claims he has a new girlfriend. There is always a lot of boasting and exaggeration.

Frank, "Did you have sex ten times last night again, George?"

George throws Frank a dirty look, whilst we all burst out laughing.

Marios, "I won one thousand dollars over the weekend." Marios only tells us of the times he wins at poker and always exaggerates the amount. The money he loses is more than the money he wins.

Frank is still miffed at the joke about his car. "I would quit my job if I were you Marios. You are the only person I know, who claims to always win at poker. I have never heard you say that you lost."

Oh! How I missed these stupid conversations.

I caught my wife's eye. She was at the other end of the room, smiling and talking to some friends of her own.

I felt that being at the party was good. Good for me and good for my wife. She could laugh and talk about something other than getting pregnant.

Out of the corner of my eye, I saw a woman reach out and hug my wife. Fifteen minutes later, my wife came over, her eyes red, saying she was not feeling well. We said our goodbyes and left.

Alone in the car, when I asked what was wrong, she offered the same excuse again, but I already knew.

"She asked if I was pregnant," she began. "When I said I wasn't, she told me she was sure I would be a mother, to which I answered, 'I hope so,' but then the tears came. I just couldn't stop crying, even as she cuddled me."

My blood boiled. Why couldn't people ever mind their own business?

Four long years later, we were at a Greek wedding. It was a typical British night: cold, rainy, and miserable, just like my mood. Since infertility had decided to stick around, anger, frustration, and depression were at an all-time high. I hoped, for a few hours at least, that my mind could occupy itself with something other than babies and ovulation charts. I thought back to when we used to laugh, have conversations with friends about silly and funny stuff, and let our hair down. I wanted to forget what was eating me up inside twenty-four hours a day. Infertility be damned! How long did we have to wait before we got a positive result? Why did this have to happen to us?

With total terror, I noticed the same woman from the party approaching my wife. From the other side of the hall, I rushed over, but a sea of people blocked the way to her. Bloody Greeks and weddings (forever mingling around and blocking all the routes). I ducked around the first person, nudged the second gently out of the way, and pushed through the remaining rabble. With dread, I witnessed the same scene unfolding. Damn it! She had already put her arms around my wife. I was too late. Vas was already in tears.

"Why did you upset my wife again?" I thundered at the woman.

"I only asked her if she is pregnant!"

By then, living with infertility had taken its toll. I was no longer the carefree and tolerant person.

"Does she look pregnant to you?" I stormed.

My wife looked mortified.

"No. I'm sure that she'll become a mom, though."

"No kidding! Why don't you tell us how you know this so we can stop feeling sorry for ourselves?"

"I don't know for sure, but I sincerely hope so."

The idiocy of that statement had me ready to explode.

"You hope so? I don't care to listen to what you hope for!"

The woman's mouth fell open.

"Do you know why we came here? We were hoping to occupy our minds with something else. You have just brought us back to the place we have been desperately trying to escape."

"Sorry. I didn't mean to upset you."

"You did though," I replied with now-uncontrollable anger. "Look at my wife. She is trying to hold it together, but she can't. Next time before you open your mouth, make sure you don't cause distress to other people." I went in for the kill. "Thank you for ruining our evening."

Unashamedly turning my back to her, I took my wife's hand and, together, we left the wedding. It was still cold and wet. I felt as if smoke was coming out of my ears. Instead of being happy for the newlyweds, all I wanted was to inflict pain on that woman with the big mouth.

Have you lived with infertility? Has it taken over your life to the point that nothing else matters?

Do you yearn for a baby so much that you think about nothing else? In your anger, have you spoken cruel words to anyone?

My story is not just about infertility. I thought living with infertility was tough. It is. Little did I know, though, that I had a date with death, terror, and madness!

Has your wife suffered a miscarriage, or have you lost a baby because of a birth defect?

You may be in the mall or taking a solitary walk when you see a parent screaming like crazy at her/his tearful and terrified baby. Instead of loving, guiding, nurturing, and being thankful for achieving this miracle, they behave in a manner you wouldn't. Did you think they didn't deserve to have children? Did you want to grab them by the throat? Were you positive that there is no justice in this world? I was immersed in all of the above. I felt I was drowning.

My struggle did not end there. It grew, and it felt as if I was on a runaway train heading straight to hell.

Have you ever spoken harshly to your wife because she was willing to make you a widower? Did you ever reach a stage where your only function was keeping score of the dead and barely alive members of your family and all you could see was a future of nothingness? Worse yet, have you ever received a call from your wife and all you could hear was her panic, fear, desperation, and helplessness, making you lose the will to live? I have!

The thing is, I only wanted to be a dad. I did not expect what was coming my way.

I believe the noblest of dreams is to create life. A person can achieve, through hard work a healthy bank balance and a portfolio of properties, but they all fade into insignificance when you compare it with creating life. Having a child to nurture, guide, and love will bring you unimaginable happiness and completeness.

This was our dream, which became my living nightmare.

Where we were hopeful, we were terror stricken.

Where we wanted to create life, we encountered death.

My story started with my wife's desire to become a mom. She wanted to create life.

This is not an imaginary story where, at the end, the hero gallops away into the sunset with music blaring in the background.

This is my true-life story, and I doubt it'll leave audiences feeling warm and fuzzy.

I didn't get to determine how my story ended. There was no galloping away—only death. Instead of music, alarms rang out. Despair, hate, and anger were all I was capable of feeling, for I lost my humanity.

If there are heroes in my story, they are my wife, the world's mothers, and every woman who tried and didn't achieve this noble dream. Some of these women carry the scars of their experiences to their dying days

This is only one man's story-- the story of how I handled (or, more appropriately, didn't handle) myself when faced with problems along the way.

CHAPTER ONE

ABOUT ME AND 'I ONLY WANTED TO BE A DAD.'

"I have no business, being in the book world. Just fish and chips."

There are four things that define me:

      *I am committed, dedicated, and relentless.

      *I have regrets.

      This book is the sequel to *All I Ever Wanted Was to Be Called Mom*, which I have written with my wife. It is our true life story. I wrote most of *AIEWWTBCM*, as my wife found it difficult to relive those harrowing times. It was quite therapeutic—I was a man on a mission. The writing continued even after I exceeded the recommended number of words. Reviewing it a second time, made me realize that I had been digressing from the main theme of the book. Yes, I was dealing with my demons, but they had no place in the first book. Large segments were then taken out, which you will find in this book.

Although we had been through a terrible ordeal, there were many reasons to keep our suffering private. At the time, the whole experience was so intense, and with Vas being hospitalized, it was up to me to provide information and updates to our nearest and dearest. Since the experience turned me into an antisocial monster, by default, I wasn't in a communicative mood.

In the following years, there were a few attempts between us to discuss it. Each time it happened, Vas broke down in tears, and her nightmares intensified. Yes, we had lived to tell the tale, but we were not prepared to relive that period of our lives just yet.

I put it out of my mind. The way I saw it was that since we had somehow survived our nightmare, we might as well let sleeping dogs lie. Why disturb the hornet's nest when there is no need to do so? Apart from Vas's nightmares, we never regarded ourselves as mentally affected. We got on with our lives.

Writing a book about it might seem extreme, but I felt we had something to share. Despite my wife's reluctance to unearth bad memories, she participated, and I'm so proud of her. Sharing your thoughts and feelings about the most frightening periods of your life is a difficult mountain to climb, but climb we did, hand-in-hand. We started as a unit, and we shall finish as one to our dying days. This is who we are.

We are VASPX

While writing these books, I became surprisingly emotional. Those who know me can confirm that I show little emotion. You never realize how damaged you are until you deal with your demons. I had put a lid on hate, despair, grieving, and helplessness. With the lid removed, feelings I never thought I was capable of expressing surfaced, overwhelming me.

I am a fish and chips shop owner/operator. The title of 'cook' is more appropriate than 'author.' I cook barrels of chips and boxes of fish on a daily basis but can't even boil an egg. I'm five-foot-nine. Whereas some people have what looks like a rainforest on their heads, my own scalp is more like a scattered deforestation; thus kept shaved. I am quite lazy by nature which always baffles me — why did I choose to run this kind of business? Unsociable hours and hard work. Ah well, at least it gives me considerable free time to write.

I was born in Cyprus (Greek-Cypriot) and am now living in England. Greek is my first language. If you heard me talk, you would question whether it was really me who wrote this book. A word like 'sword,' I pronounce using all the letters, as we do in Greek.

If you have seen the film *My Big Fat Greek Wedding*, picture me speaking like the old characters.

I've learned many things while writing these books.

Chief among them: editing your own book is a tough process. You don't have the heart to remove things. You are biased. Editing your true-life story is even more difficult. Every time I decide to remove something, I feel as if my arm will fall off. I feel guilty and try to conjure up a myriad of excuses as to why I shouldn't delete a particular sequence. It can sometimes drive me nuts.

That is why I prefer cooking fish and chips to writing. It is so much easier! A friend of mine, Ken from Minnesota (who likes cooking), read our first book. He liked the book very much. In his review[1], he rightly said that I am a fish and chips owner/operator first and an author second. I guess he wanted to encourage people to keep keep reading, even if the going got tough. For this, I'm grateful.

---

[1] You can read Ken's full review on his website: http://toptenbookreview.com

CHAPTER TWO

<u>HOW IT STARTED FOR US</u>

"Hope and optimism were rife."

Vas agreed to spend the rest of her life with me, and we got married. I knew I had married wisely! Soon after, we decided to try for a baby. This was the beginning of Vas's dream, and I was going along for the ride. I was indifferent at the time—truth be told, I'd never had that yearning. If it happened, it happened. If it didn't happen, then it was no big deal.

Vas was excited and told everyone. I thought nothing of it at the time—what difference could it make? We lived through the first few months grinning and planning, as most people do. For the unlucky ones, the grins turn quickly to frowns, and the planning turns into depression.

The bottom line is that Vas should have kept quiet about us trying to get pregnant. I believe that every couple should do this, and not say anything until the woman gets past the first three months of pregnancy. No one knows how they will fare once they embark on this journey. We all hope we shall sail through it, but as we know all too well, life is not full of roses for everyone. For the unlucky ones, this period is hell.

Trying to get pregnant can sometimes take years. It can be a long, painful, stressful, and angry time. This period can test the strength of your marriage, even when just you and your wife know of your problem. If you share your plans and do face problems, prepare for friends and relatives to repeatedly ask 'the question.'

The more you try to minimize intrusions during this rollercoaster period, the better. What kind of support can friends and loved ones really provide? Unless they've had the same problems, all you will get are the clichéd words, "You will be alright. I am sure you will get pregnant." What else can they give you?

In the beginning, after fussing over a baby, Vas would be in tears. Whoever was there would try to reassure her that her turn would come.

There were a lot of tears over the years. Seeing my wife so upset made me rearrange our lives, trying to avoid meeting people we knew were pregnant or had a baby. Since all our friends had at least one baby, our social life dried up. I always claimed that we couldn't go somewhere because the shop was busy.

I don't regret it — it was the only way we could have

coped. There was nothing to be gained by going out. It was killing me seeing my wife sad. Witnessing a whispered conversation that would suddenly stop when we approached made my blood boil. The precious few times we went out was to forget, and those people were pushing us back to the hellhole we were trying to escape from.

Plenty of times, the question, "It is about time you have a baby, don't you think?" ruined our evening out at a function or dinner. Their sheer stupidity and ignorance infuriated me. It was as if they thought we were actually going out of our way not to get pregnant so as not to ruin our social life. We had no social life! My response swiftly became an intense glare. They would make their excuses and leave. Then there were those with their screaming kids in tow telling us we were lucky not to have kids. "They cost a fortune, and they are full of tantrums." These people were even worse.

One year went by, and Vas still didn't become pregnant. Sex became a casualty, happening not when I wanted but when Vas told me she was ovulating. Up until then, I'd thought the best time to have sex was when we were both horny. These were the 'puppet times.'

By this time, Vas would rarely smile. She would stay in her room for hours at a time. I felt useless—there was nothing I could do to help her. My best simply wasn't enough. Inside me,

I bottled up my frustration.

What was left for us to do? Go out one night, get drunk, have sex when we got home, and pray for pregnancy? It seemed to work for everyone else. Sadly, I am not much of a drinker. When I have a few drinks, the only thing that seems to work is my mouth. Drinking does not inspire the *general*.

We both made sacrifices. I like to sometimes smoke cigars, but that little pleasure had to stop—apparently, it could affect the performance of my swimmers. The same happened with malt whiskey.

Complete surrender!

We both felt terribly lonely. If you are unlucky and you have to live with this struggle for a few years, it can be quite demoralizing. I still loved my wife, and we were still communicating, but sadness had slipped into our lives and taken root. I saw my wife at her lowest. I was tiptoeing around her, trying not to cause her unnecessary distress. I felt I could not tell her exactly how I felt, for I was afraid it would make her feel even worse.

Meanwhile, our friends got pregnant and had babies. We were caught in a loop, and I could see no way out of it.

This is what was constantly going through my mind, "What *the hell is wrong with us? Why did this have to happen to us? Stop telling us it is about time we had a baby! Stop asking us if we are pregnant! You cannot possibly understand what we are going through! Leave us alone!"*

An overweight woman (or man), may stop going out so that she will not have to endure people staring at her. In the prison of her home, when watching television, she will be bombarded with adverts and shows with skinny people smiling. She cannot escape. Whether you are bald, short, fat, have deformities, health issues, you cannot escape the torture. It will find you. Infertility is one of them.

When I went home, I often found my wife in tears. In the beginning, I would cuddle her and ask what was wrong. With time, I stopped asking. I could hear her talking on the phone and then only the sobbing. With time, I always tried to answer the phone. She would lash out at me, and I would sometimes naively try to explain to her why I believed it was unreasonable. With time, I learned to stay quiet and keep my head down.

CHAPTER THREE

<u>INFERTILITY</u>

"Infertility does not discriminate against color, race, or wealth."

You will notice that the first part of the book revolves around infertility and rightly so. I want to highlight the problem as it is the cause for derailing your plans and your future. When infertility makes its presence known, the couple will find out that their life as they know it is over. It is the first signal that tough times lay ahead. This monster decided to stick around and brought nothing but misery and depression in our lives. It made every year feel like a decade.

What is infertility?

According to the American Infertility Association: "Infertility is a disease that results in the abnormal functioning of the male or female reproductive system."[2]

One in eight couples faces problems getting pregnant or achieving pregnancy. This *affects about 7.0 million couples in the USA.*

---

[2] See www.resolve.com

According to the English Infertility Association[3], one in six couples has problems becoming parents. This affects about 3.5 million couples in the UK.

In Australia, more than one in six couples has problems. It's the same in Russia.[4] In India, there are 20 million infertile couples.[5] It's twice that in China.[6]

The figures are quite sobering, are they not?

It is not enough to just hear the ratio of one in eight. The actual numbers put things into grim perspective.

The World Health Organization forecasted that 48.5 million couples worldwide would suffer from infertility by 2010. We are now in 2018 and, irrespective of the increase in the Earth's population, the number of infertile couples is rising.

Today, there are between fifty to eighty million couples who live this nightmare, full of frustration, depression, and anger.

In the old days, people prayed to their gods and made sacrifices so that they would be blessed with a baby. When they couldn't conceive, they blamed themselves for displeasing the

[3] See www.infertilitynetworkuk.com

[4] See http://www.nhs.uk/Conditions/Infertility/Pages/Introduction.aspx

[5] See http://www.thehindu.com/sunday-anchor/pushpa-m-bhargava-there-are-20-million-infertile-couples-in-india/article6453374.ece

[6] See www.forbes.com/sites/.../2012/.../chinas-one-child-policys-unexpected-issue-infertility

gods.

It is no better today. Some people see it as a stigma; they see it as their own personal failing. It is not. It is a random and cruel illness that intrudes into people's lives and brings devastation in its wake.

Ordinary people and celebrities alike suffer from this. Nobody is safe.

Celebrities guard their privacy ferociously. Imagine one of them living through the torture of infertility with the media splashing it on the front pages of tabloids. It would be torture on an epic scale, for the world would know their struggle. Wherever they went, it would be the first thing they'd be questioned on. Would you blame them if they keep quiet about having lived with infertility and IVF?

It was encouraging to see several celebrities talk openly about their personal experiences with the monster of infertility. Their sharing helped other people to open up. Having already publicly spoken about it, I am sure they will not be offended if I mention some of them: Nicole Kidman, Celine Dion, Courtney Cox, Sarah Jessica Parker, and Nia Vardalos—you are a shining example to us all. They had the grace to be open about such a private ordeal, and at the time, they probably walked the red carpet with sad smiles on their faces. Despite all their money and influence, infertility paid them a visit. Some of them never managed to give birth. Hugh Jackman had spoken about it as well.

Coming back to us ordinary people; you have possibly met up with friends and had a sad smile on your face, pretending everything is fine. You never let on about your struggle. You most probably thought it was only you suffering at the hands of this monster. It is not. Tens of millions have to endure this pain. You are not alone.

Infertility does not just happen to ordinary people. It does not discriminate against color, race, or class. It reduces you to someone who merely watches as others continue their lives — you remain marooned at the point it made its presence known.

Picture this: it is a glorious morning with a bright blue sky. The birds are chirping their delightful melodies, and you can smell the intoxicating aroma of the flowers. Looking around, you feel blessed and thankful for witnessing such a magnificent spectacle. For an infertile couple, the effect is different. For them, it might as well be six feet of snow or torrential rain. Nothing else matters to them apart from having a baby. Until they manage to have a baby (if they do at all), there is nothing but emptiness in their lives.

Couples who have never had to struggle for pregnancy might not understand this feeling. Living with infertility catches you in a loop. Every month, you try to get pregnant, and then the 'period' appears, month after month and year after year. In the beginning, you are positive and hopeful. Living with this problem for a few years, however, can knock the optimism out of you. Disappointment, helplessness, and anger are rife. Your life is in limbo.

You must have seen a film where the clouds speed up, people blur, and time hurries on. Within seconds, you get to see the change in seasons, buildings knocked down or built, and life going on. Every aspect of life follows the unstoppable tide of time moving forward. Well, except for infertile couples. They just exist in that specific time forever — their lives cannot possibly move forward.

One day, I took Vas to 'Petrous', one of Gordon Ramsay's restaurants in London. I hoped that for a few hours she would forget. She did forget for about ten minutes after I joked that we should sue him for using our surname as the name of his restaurant. But soon, she began to play with her food. An aura of melancholy seemed to emanate from her. She couldn't care less whether she was there eating a posh meal or having beans on toast at home. Nothing, absolutely nothing else mattered. I think she actually wished she was at home.

When I first met Vas, I kept telling her jokes, which she found hilarious. I always delivered them with a deadpan face. I probably only know about twenty! Whenever we were together or on the phone, we were always laughing. It was a happy atmosphere, and I thought it would continue forever. Infertility took that away from us. It was hard for me, seeing her smile disappear and not hearing her laughter. I thought I could fix that. I tried to repeat jokes I'd heard with pitiful results. I tried so many times that I got on her nerves. The more she didn't like them, the more I tried to invent new ones. I am not a comedian. I suck at telling jokes. I kept trying because I was so desperate to put a smile on her face.

We all try to create life, thinking that it will be easy. No one expects infertility to happen to them. We think that it is something that happens to other people. I didn't expect it either, but to my horror, I found out I was in the club of one in eight. The change in attitude can be overwhelming.

As a man, you may start by thinking your wife will fall pregnant easily because of your glorious performance in bed. When you are forced to face ovulation charts and, horror of horrors, the prospect that you've been firing blanks the whole time, you can retreat into yourself.

More and more couples face problems with infertility. It could be:

- The problem resides with the woman.

- The problem resides with the man.

- The problem remains undiagnosed.

- The problem resides in age.

Confronting the true reason can be quite daunting, but at least it gives you something to focus on. It allows you to hope again; to hope that, as soon as that specific problem is put right, you will, at last, have a decent chance of getting pregnant. Suppose that your test results revealed nothing that could explain your inability to get pregnant — there would be no obstacle to focus on. You will feel like banging your head against the wall.

Some give up while others seek help from their doctor, but this is no guarantee of success. They will most probably live with the raw pain the rest of their lives.

Others will continue to fight the good fight and will embark on IVF with still no guarantee of success beyond a heavily bruised bank balance and a tormented wife.

You must have heard at least one person say, "I'm not ready to have a baby yet. I'm going to focus on my career first or wait until I save some money/get that promotion/buy a house." They feel they have time and are confident that it will definitely happen when they are ready. Years go by and, unknown to them, time is ticking away. The quality of the sperm/egg is degrading.

Here comes the kicker. The promotion, money, and house will mean nothing. They would be willing to give it all up in a heartbeat, but alas, they can't.

It is fine if they are not one in eight, but if they are, and infertility decides to stick around, they will find out the hard way that what they wish for and what they get might be two different things.

Some people suffering from infertility have another torment to live with. Regrets! "If only I hadn't drunk so much in my younger days or hadn't tried those recreational drugs. If only I had adopted a better diet or wasn't so sexually active ..." The list is endless.

Living with infertility does not end there. You will find out that your desperation is so great that you will be willing to try anything, however far-fetched it is. A friend of Vas's sent her a fertility doll. It was supposed to bring luck to infertile women. Looking at it objectively, it's nonsense. My wife kept it next to her side of the bed, hoping it would do its magic.

All this heartache from trying to create life. All this devastation from a start full of dreams and hope.

I connected on Twitter with Mrs Kelly Da Silva (@thedovecoteorg). She wanted to be a mother. Instead, she battled infertility and then attempted IVF. She had four attempts with sadly no result. She was devastated. She knew that that was the end of her journey as far as having a baby was concerned. She knew that she now faced a childless future. She had counseling, she cried and she mourned. Eventually, she emerged from her dark place with a new resolve and purpose in life.

This warrior princess, who shines in her selfless efforts to help others dealing with a childless future, is the founder of 'The Dovecote'[7]. The Dovecote is an organisation established to enable people facing involuntary childlessness to obtain support, strategies, knowledge and experiences to discover a renewed life of passion and purpose."

Selfless and dedicated! She said this in an article in the Mirror[8], "I spend so many years making excuses about not having them. I won't be ashamed anymore." I felt a chill down my spine when I read that.

When I meet people like Kelly, I feel that this is truly a cruel and unjust world.

You must have seen on telly the devastation a hurricane leaves behind or when a reporter gives his first impression after visiting a place plagued by war. Buildings left in tatters, kids crying and people having that empty look in their eyes. This is how a woman feels when she is facing a childless future.

Damn infertility and the baggage it brings with it.

---

[7]http://www.thedovecote.org

[8]http://www.mirror.co.uk/news/real-life-stories/after-years-heartbreak-ive-finally-7904568?ICID=facebook_instant_phF

CHAPTER FOUR

<u>TWO CHOICES WHEN YOU DECIDE</u> <u>TO TRY TO GET PREGNANT</u>

"Keep quiet and when you get pregnant, shout it from the rooftops."

From my blog: www.vaspx.com

Trying to get pregnant is one of the biggest decisions a couple can make. Deciding to bring a life into the world, for which they will be responsible for nurturing and guiding, is daunting and awesome at the same time.

When the decision is made, they have two choices:

1. Keep it to themselves.

2. Share it with friends and family.

If they keep it to themselves and get pregnant straight away, there's no harm done. If they have trouble getting pregnant, they suffer in silence and continue trying while everyone around them is clueless to their anguish and torment. They have no outside pressure, as no one is any the wiser.

If they share their plans with others and get pregnant straight away, again, no harm done. However, here comes the kicker… if they have trouble getting pregnant, they will not only have to put up with their own private hell but also with intrusions from their nearest and dearest.

The last thing you need if you are fruitlessly trying to get pregnant is friends and relatives asking you every month if you are pregnant yet or putting their arms around you and telling you it will be all right. It is bad enough dealing with your own depressing inability to get pregnant without having them ask you every single month, reminding you of your failure. Your problem is amplified. You don't need this unnecessary pressure. You will get more quality support by going on the Internet and following blogs or joining groups that deal with infertility. These people share their journeys, and you can interact with them — these are people in the same 'club' as you. You are more likely to receive understanding from strangers who are going through what you are going through than from friends and relatives. This is why I stress repeatedly that the fewer people that know, the better.

When you are finally pregnant, shout it from the rooftops. Before you reach that stage, though, keep it to yourself if you can help it.

"Don't worry! I just know it will happen for you!" How many times have you heard these empty words from friends and relatives?

Did you feel like banging your head (or their head!) against the wall? By voicing these clichéd words, they feel they have done their duty to be supportive towards you. They then get on with the rest of their day while you are still seething about their lack of understanding. Imagine the difference if you hadn't told them about trying to get pregnant? You would still have to face this daunting problem, but with fewer intrusions and upsetting conversations from your nearest and dearest.

Every time the pitying looks and whispers re-emerge, you will tense up. When you go home, your wife will be in tears as anger and depression kick in. You could have avoided all this. Too many things can go wrong with this endeavour, so the fewer people that know, the better. This is my humble opinion.

We suffered. We fought to achieve our miracle. We are **VASPX**.

CHAPTER FIVE

LIVING WITH INFERTILITY

"Infertility has been around forever. It was here yesterday, it is here today, and it will most certainly raise its ugly head tomorrow."

From my blog: www.vaspx.com

Living with infertility for a few years grants you the privilege of experiencing problems and emotions previously inconceivable. You deal with things that never previously crossed your mind. Infertility adds another dynamic to any relationship, regardless of its security, that was never part of the equation in the first place. Infertility can break a marriage. This is how bad the problem is.

It had a huge effect on my wife and myself. I was walking on eggshells around my wife, as I was afraid that whatever I said or did, I would get on her nerves. I began to feel like a puppet when asked to perform, as ovulation charts and temperature plotting took over the bedroom. My wife endured intense mood swings and depression as she tried desperately to fulfil her dream of being a mother, feeling more and more like a It had a huge effect on my wife and myself. I was walking on eggshells around my wife, as I was afraid that whatever I said or did, I would get on her nerves. I began to feel like a puppet when asked to perform, as ovulation charts and temperature plotting took over the bedroom. My wife endured intense mood swings and depression as she tried desperately to fulfil her dream of being a mother, feeling more and more like a failure. Behind her tough exterior lay a tortured and fragile soul who needed understanding and compassion. Behind my supportive shell lay a confused and lost man.

Gone were the sexy weekends away, long lie-ins, and spontaneous trips to the bedroom. Now everything was organised, planned, and prepared. I had to be ready to perform on command.

There were many times when I would get home and find my wife in tears. I just cuddled her. I never asked her why. I knew! I never told her that we were going to be alright and that our turn to be parents would come. It was bad enough hearing this from our nearest and dearest. When you have nothing constructive to say, silence is the best option.

I am a social drinker and a smoker. Just like that, those little pleasures were gone. My diet changed. As the years passed and still nothing happened, I questioned the wisdom of those little sacrifices. What if after five or ten years of trying, we still didn't get a result? What if all this was for nothing? What if…?

I never voiced any of this to my wife. How could I?

This was when the resentment started to surface. *Was my wife's need to be a mother worth the daily hassles we were going through? How long would I have to put up with her mood swings and depression? Our lives were in limbo. Why could we not cut our losses and finally start getting on with our lives? We could have still lived a productive life without children! There had been no laughter in our house for five years. Surely, enough was enough.*

To my shame, I thought about all these things, but thankfully, I never voiced them. I never realised how deep that desire ran. My wife felt like less of a woman. She felt ashamed! Her not being able to be a mom made her question the reason for her existence.

To be honest, I would have followed her on this road until the end. We would have been seventy years old, boxes full of Viagra, still trying! This was her battle and, by default, it became my battle.

When you embark on this journey, and you face problems, the things that will see you through are communication, understanding, compassion, faith, and love for each other. You need to face this battle as a unit, without allocating blame.

In my opinion, living with infertility is nothing more than being in prison. I was stuck there, not being able to think about anything else. There were limitations as to what I could drink and eat. I stopped going out and meeting friends and family who had kids or were pregnant. I became a prisoner in my own home. And, just like in prison where guards or other inmates intrude into your solitude, we had the busybodies calling to see if Vas was pregnant.

We suffered. We fought to achieve our miracle. We are VASPX.

CHAPTER SIX

<u>SECONDARY INFERTILITY</u>

Why do I call infertility a monster? Because no one is safe.

Suppose that a couple got pregnant easily and they had their first baby. Without giving it a second thought, when they think that they are ready, they try for a second baby. Of course, they think it will be as easy as the first time. Why shouldn't they?

Six or so months down the line, there is still no 'result'. They continue trying, baffled, frustrated and angry as to why it is not working for them this time.

They will go to their doctor for a consultation and advice.

It's still not working.

A year has passed and they are now classed as suffering from secondary infertility.

'Secondary infertility' is the inability to get pregnant or carry a baby to full term after previously giving birth to a baby.

There is not a lot of data available on secondary infertility but according to Kims Cuddles[9], in America there are about three million women suffering from this.

When they realise they can't get pregnant again, they will stillface similar pressures like most infertile couples. The pain doesn't go away because they already have a baby. They still have that yearning. They will go back to basics like temperature plotting and ovulation charts. If that fails they will then try IVF.

As a man suffering from primary infertility, how would I've reacted upon hearing of a couple's plight who was suffering from secondary infertility?

- They are so selfish.
- They already have a baby.
- They are just seeking attention.
- Once they relax, it will happen for them, unlike us who suffer from the real monster of infertility.
- They haven't got a clue about what it means to suffer from infertility.

This is how I would have reacted back in the day. Now my view is different.

As I grow older and having had the benefit of my life experiences; compassion and understanding are second nature for me.

What do couples go through when coming face to face with secondary infertility?

---

[9] https://www.kimscuddles.com/causes-of-secondary-infertility/

* They face stress and frustration like anyone else trying to get pregnant.

* The fact that they are already parents doesn't make it easier. They don't just get over it. They are not selfish by wanting more babies.

* They still have to face hurtful questions from their nearest and dearest.

* They might feel guilty for wanting another baby, when there are millions who can't have even one.

* They'll not just relax and it will happen for them.

Some probable causes of secondary infertility:

- Complications relating to previous pregnancy. An injury to the uterus or fallopian tube might make it more difficult to get pregnant again.

-Impaired sperm production in relation to men.

- Fibroids. Abnormal growths that develop on or inside the uterus. They can develop or worsen after pregnancy.

-Age. When there is a big time gap between the first pregnancy and the current attempt. The later you leave it to get pregnant, the less your chances are.

The bottom line is, whether you have a baby or not, you may still get a visit from the monster of infertility.

CHAPTER SEVEN

<u>I WAS THE KING!</u>

"I am flawed. Trying desperately to learn from my mistakes."

Do you remember the king from the fable who paraded naked before his subjects, thinking that he was wearing a cloak which it turned out was invisible to those who were stupid, incompetent, or otherwise unfit for duty? If you believe that he was stupid, he was quite clever compared to me.

There will be a bit of swearing further on, for which I apologise. However, this will grant a more realistic vision of my distress during that period, for it was full of profanity. Cleansing the book of such words will not redeem my actions. In any case, this is a very much edited account. Were an unedited version presented, you definitely would dismiss me as a lost soul.

The funny thing is, though, I was never like that. I am not looking for sympathy here; I am not trying to justify my actions. But never have I felt despair and helplessness like that in my whole life. A few swear words are nothing compared to the anger and hate I felt towards you. Yes, you. I didn't know you existed, but I still hated you, for you could have been happy at the time I was drowning. That was the depth of my failure as a human being. Yes, for that I really am sorry.

I hope you'll agree that a few swear words are nothing compared to being the king!

When you are promoted to king, you don't at first realise the transformation. You change, but you still think you are the same person. You become a jerk with the audacity to think that everyone around you is an idiot and that you are the only sane person around. If I could go back in time, I would've given myself a well-earned slap and a good telling off, for I deserved it.

Wherever you see '*I was the king!*' it is the indicator when I acknowledge that I did something wrong.

CHAPTER EIGHT

<u>SEX AND INFERTILITY</u>
"No two-hour sex marathon! No angels weeping. Just bloody

puppet-times."

Sex is a very important and pleasurable activity in an average man's life. A widely-held belief is that a man thinks about sex every seven seconds.

When you are a young man, you think about and try to have sex at every opportunity. It is the main issue in your life at the time.

When you first try to get pregnant, it is as if it is Christmas every day. He feels he is a stud. He is 'The Man.'

For most married men, their wives get pregnant within a reasonable timeframe. For some of us, this is not the case. Years go by and still nothing. Irrespective of how many times and how often you perform, your swimmers never conquer the motherland. You try to give your best performance, falsely thinking that you are in control. How far from the truth that is!

I have already talked about ovulation charts and temperature plotting. The truth is, you begin to hate sex! The pleasure has left the building!

Irrespective of how you feel, when you go home (if she is

ovulating), she will expect you to perform at a moment's notice.

Imagine having a shitty day at work. Maybe someone's made you angry. You get home still spitting feathers about what happened. As soon as you open the front door, your wife is there waiting for you. She tells you in a businesslike tone to come to the bedroom as she is at her optimum time of ovulation. All you wanted was to come home, have a stiff drink, and moan to your wife about the jerk that pissed you off at work. Obviously, you dare not say that you don't feel like it, and instead, hope that the *general* will find it in his heart to rise to the occasion, as your mind can't be trusted — it's still angry from work. If the *general* declines, a barrage of recriminations arrives.

"Don't you want to have a baby?"

"Don't you love me?"

"Don't you find me sexy anymore?"

Unbelievable! All the things you want to say but dare not.

Like: *"Of course I bloody love you. That is why I married you. I am just pissed off tonight! Okay?"*

It happened quite a few times with us. I never complained or refused. With a stiff upper lip, I performed as needed. It was not how I'd imagined our sex life would be. It reduced sex to just another task I had to complete. This desire of my wife's so consumed her that my feelings went ignored. *I was the king!*

The other side of the coin is equally tough: when you are finally horny, and you start going through the motions, she tells you in a matter-of-fact way that she will be ovulating in two days, and that you must wait until then.

Gone are the long weekends that you used to go on with your wife to rekindle your love for each other.

Gone are the times when you could have a celebratory cigar after a glorious performance. *I was the king!*

They say that sex is not the most important factor in keeping a marriage alive, and rightly so. Love, understanding, communication, and compassion make the marriage. Sex is still there, though. A man still needs those two hours (or more appropriately those two minutes!). If it takes years to get pregnant, let me assure you they can feel like decades — you start living vicariously through your friends. When they exaggerate about their conquests, you smile, never letting on you are no longer in that happy club. You start reliving the fond memories of those early days of carefree sex with your wife at the beginning and wonder where it all went wrong. *I was the king!*

There can be no more whispering of sweet nothings in her ear. There is no more play-acting.

There is just clinical sex.

Women will be in uproar when they read what I write next, and yet, here it is: *You feel cheap! You feel used!*

That is right. You read it correctly. But remember: *I was the king!*

Sometimes I was angry at Vas because of our clinical sex life. I never voiced it, as I didn't want to upset her. I actually thought that I was being an understanding husband. The truth is, that was my first lie to her and my second wrong step. *I was the king!*

Well ...

You've decided that you are mature enough to try to have a baby.

When you want to buy a car, you will spend hours/days/weeks searching on the internet. The color, horsepower, alloy wheels, sensors, service history, finance ... the list is endless. If you are willing to invest so much time to learn about a car, failure to put in the time to learn and understand the possible problems relating to infertility will be your first wrong step.

As a man, I believe you have a responsibility always to be there for your wife.

The very first thing that you (and I) should learn is how deep that desire to become a mother runs.

Imagine that you are impotent and see your wife harmlessly talking and laughing with another man. That man can be your neighbor, colleague, friend, or even some stranger asking her for directions.

You will tense and at the same time have overwhelming doubts,

"He's trying to get my wife to bed!"

"It's only a matter of time before she leaves me for a real man."

You feel inadequate, and despite the reassuring words she gives you, your feelings that cuddling her is all you are good for and inadequacy consume you. You lost your manhood, willing to go to any lengths to get it back.

Becoming a mom is your wife's womanhood. Every time you have sex, and every time she is late with her period, she will be hopeful and praying. Month after month, year after year, her period will appear taunting her:

"You're a failure as a woman. You'll never become a mom."

When she goes shopping, she will see pregnant women or mothers with their babies. Your friends and family will call with their good news that they are pregnant. The same ones will be asking her if she is pregnant. Even something as harmless as watching a film can upset her, for it is bound to have a pregnant woman or babies. When you go to a christening or a baby's birthday, it has the same effect. For your wife, infertility is non-stop torture. If she cannot be a mother, then what is the point of it all? Do you now understand how deep her need runs?

The final torment she might be feeling is, "How long is he going to stick around? Why is he still with me? He will most probably leave me soon, for a real woman who can have his baby!"

Imagine her battling infertility and having these doubts about you! She needs reassurance, understanding, and total commitment. It is not enough for you knowing that you are committed to her. She is not a mind reader. Tell her and keep telling her every day. She needs to hear those words coming from you, more than you know. Do this, and it will show to her that she has married wisely.

Now that you understand, you can face this problem with more sympathy and compassion towards your wife.

Living through infertility may put a damper on your sex life. Accept it, and be prepared. The times that she will ask you to perform can be done with pleasure and pride, and not resentment and self-pity. By first understanding her torment, it empowers you to get closer to her, really to be a strong shoulder for her to lean on. Instead of worrying about my wife's torture and depression, I was stressing over the fact that our sex life took a nosedive. Talk about selfish! *I was the king!*

You take the first step of not understanding your wife's need, and then it is downhill from then on. Never take that first wrong step. The torment and depression my wife went through would have crushed me if I were in her place.

The sobering reality of this situation is that in trying to get pregnant, ovulation charts eventually will control sex. Going through IVF, you will get to become quite friendly with your *general*! Try to understand and accept this. Is this a big deal? Of course not. Stay the course, and don't falter. You owe this to the tormented soul who is waiting for you at home.

Not understanding and embracing the above will make you feel resentful towards your wife, and you will feel that you unjustly are suffering. The funny, sexy, interesting, and witty girl you first met is no more. She is depressed, scared, having low self-esteem, and angry. As a man, you might dread going home to that oppressive atmosphere.

Suppose after work, colleagues ask you to go for a few drinks. A female colleague, or a sexy girl at the bar, who had a few too many, in her drunken stupor finds you desirable. She makes suggestive eye contact, full of exciting possibilities. All you see is a short skirt and a low cut top. You can smell her intoxicating perfume, and you can hear her laughter beckoning you like a siren. To your surprise, she actually thinks you are attractive and funny! With regret, you remember your wife used to think that.

What do you do?

Girl …funny and laughing; wife …depressed and angry.

Girl …carefree and exciting sex; wife …ovulation charts and puppet.

You may feel that you deserve this one night of hot sex after all the years of being a puppet. You are sure your wife will not find out.

Shame on you! You have just done the unforgivable. You cheated on your wife. As you were pulling your pants up after your exciting sex session, I hope you realised something:

"Your wife is too good for you. You don't deserve to have her in your life, and you are right!"

For just one second, try to be in your wife's shoes. What would it feel like for both her body AND her husband to reject her? How horrible and lonely she must feel!

What's next?

Do you walk away from your marriage, hoping to find someone who can bear your children easier? You should have never left your wife alone in the first place.

When you first met, was this the kind of man you told her you were? Of course not! You told her that you would always be there for her.

Do you feel you are suffering unjustly? Big deal! Look at your wife, and see how depressed and tortured she feels. Grow a pair, get over it, and get on with it. Be the man that she thought she was going to spend the rest of her life with, and not the little boy who feels overwhelmed when things get tough.

If you think I am being hard for saying this, think again. Living with infertility is hard, taking its toll on you. Injustice, hate, and anger are at an all-time high. The easiest thing for you to do is to walk away. Play the field for a while, and probably marry again, with no guarantee that your next wife/partner will not have the same problem.

REPEAT!

By understanding that need and sharing your true feelings, being supportive, communicating, and loving with each other, you don't feel hard done by. By not taking the first wrong step, you never will entertain the idea of taking the worst one of walking away, which will be the ultimate betrayal to your wife.

Infertility! It has been around forever. It was here yesterday, it is here today, and it will most certainly raise its ugly head tomorrow.

It is an unexpected and unwelcome intruder in any relationship. It is bad enough facing infertility in your late twenties or thirties. It must be devastating facing it in your early twenties. You have just started in life with your wife/partner; getting a job, renting a flat and overall, inexperienced to the harsh realities of life. As a young couple full of dreams and hope, you can sometimes find this period overwhelming. It is and unfortunately this applies to whatever age bracket you are! It has split up countless couples. Don't become just another statistic.

A Danish study[10] showed that infertile couples are three times more likely to divorce.

You will live with a wife who is suffering from depression because of this. Accept this, and be there for her, for she deserves nothing less. There is no magic cure. You are no longer in control of your life. Whatever she wants you to do or try, do it because she is tortured.

The first time I saw my wife standing on her head with her legs resting on the wall, in order to help my swimmers find her eggs, I thought she lost the plot. The pain and desperation were so great that she was willing to do and try anything. She was living with them twenty-four hours a day. How she kept her sanity is beyond me.

To emphasise this point I shall tell you about something that regularly happened in our lives during infertility. My wife

---

[10] See https://www.usnews.com/news/articles/2014/01/31/study-infertile-couples-3-times-more-likely-to-divorce

would sometimes disappear in the bathroom and after ten minutes she would come out. Her eyes would be red and would sometimes tell me that she just saw her period or that she had just done a pregnancy test which was negative. I would cuddle her and tell her that it was okay. I meant it, but as the infertile years trotted along I would sometimes think in my head, "Bloody Hell, here comes another month of being a bloody puppet."

I was feeling sorry for myself. I was the king!

Unknown to me at the time, during those ten minutes all on her own, my wife would cry, feel ashamed, and wanted to bang her head on the wall. All alone in that bathroom, she would fight depression, feelings of worthlessness and the despair and terror of facing a childless future.

This book is not a platform for glorifying women. I just call it as I lived through it.

If you are facing similar struggles to mine, you now know what your wife is really going through.

You may have had children without facing infertility. Know this; had it been different, your wife would have faced what my wife and countless other women went and are still going through. The desperation to do virtually anything in order to become a mom.

You will read further on[11] what my wife was willing to do, like most women would and I hope you'll be in awe of them.

This is why when as a man, you feel unjustly suffering, you will read further on[12] what my wife was willing to do, like most women would and I hope you'll be in awe of them.

This is why when as a man, you feel unjustly suffering, you should appreciate her suffering first. This will open your eyes and hopefully enable you to realize that your suffering is nothing compared to hers. Instead, be thankful and do right by her.

---

[12] See chapter 11

CHAPTER NINE

<u>FIRING BLANKS</u>

"Why should she stay with me if I am the reason that she cannot achieve her dream?"

Previously, I mentioned impotency as a means of understanding a woman's need to be a mother. Firing blanks is just as effective.

I would like to think that every man thinks like me on this one. We all think we are studs, completely satisfying our wives after our marathon lovemaking sessions. We congratulate the *general* for a job well done and want a nice cigar afterwards.

Deep down, we know that it is not true. Women know that it's not true too. The hour-long marathon probably only lasted two minutes.

Our wives are probably thinking: *This is so boring! He finished early again. He will have that stupid grin on his face and will be snoring soon! If he dares say that he fancies smoking a cigar, I shall scream (well, this is what I guess my wife thinks).*

Remember, men think differently than women. We can be quite delusional as far as sex is concerned. Well, I am.

You are trying to get pregnant. If there is a problem, the first thing you will think as a man is that the problem lies with your wife. Your general is standing proud and firing on all cylinders. Surely, the problem cannot possibly be with you. You don't even entertain the idea, for this is how clueless men are. Well, it was certainly how clueless I was.

My wife felt ashamed for being unable to get pregnant. I told her on numerous occasions that she had nothing to be ashamed of. Infertility is a random and cruel illness and she had nothing to be ashamed of. Did it help? I don't think so, but I kept telling her that nonetheless.

A year after we started our battle with infertility, a thought crossed my mind and lodged itself there, tormenting me and refusing to go away. What if the reason Vas was not getting pregnant was me? What if, even after my lion-like performance, I'd just been firing blanks? What if I could not give her what every other man can give to his wife? It was a shock to the system to admit to myself that this scenario could be real. It never crossed my mind until I saw a film where a man was firing blanks. It was so boring, I don't even remember its title. The only reason I kept watching was that the remote was on the other side of the settee. Bloody film! From that day on, that niggling thought never left my mind. It terrified me, making me feel less of a man.

When these thoughts take center stage in your mind, you

get a glimpse of a fraction of the daily torment your wife is undergoing. I never spoke about it with anyone—even the thought of sharing it made me shudder. You'd need to put a gun to my head. You see, it was then and only then that I began to walk in Vas's shoes. From then on, every time we saw babies, we both lapsed into a tense silence. Vas was silent because she felt a failure who could not get pregnant, and I was because I knew that Vas would be upset (to say nothing of that niggling possibility that Vas's inability to get pregnant was because of me). Welcome to my world!

I felt depressed and worthless. My fear and pride prevented me from doing the right thing: getting checked. *I was the king!*

I had a conversation one night with three other guys. One of them mentioned a person whom I didn't know who was firing blanks.

First idiot: "He is a half-man."

Second idiot: "Haha! I know."

Third idiot: "Who are you talking about?"

Fourth idiot is very quiet.

First idiot: "If his wife wants a baby, she should come to me."

Second idiot: "I can have a go as well."

First three idiots: "Haha!"

Fourth idiot is still quiet.

The third idiot is still not sure: "Who is the half-man then?"

First idiot: "It's Chris, you dummy."

Third idiot feels inspired: "I don't know why his wife is still with him. I'm single, available, and firing on all cylinders."

More laughter from the first three idiots but only a forced smile on the face of the fourth idiot.

Fourth idiot: "I have to go."

He abruptly disappears.

I was the fourth idiot.

I didn't have the guts to tell them to shut up. It was bad enough the poor man had to live with this torture without these three ignorant idiots making fun of him.

I was worse than they were for not speaking up. Normally, I am not one for mockery or cruelty, but they'd caught me off guard. With my tail between my legs, I retreated like a coward.

That night, they'd been laughing at Chris. I was sure that I would have been next on their list if they'd known that I was firing blanks. It was a horrible night.

Where men are concerned, locker room talk never disappears. When our wives are present, we talk about neutral, safe topics, but when they are not, we talk about how lucky women would be to spend a couple of hours with us. Pure boasting, delusion, and exaggeration. I am more of a listener, so I tend not to contribute. Worrying about firing blanks was more than enough for me to deal with!

Until I realized that I might be the problem, I had not been bothered about whether there was anything wrong with Vas. By this, I mean that if it turned out there was something wrong with her that made her incapable of having children, I would have stood by her and explored other avenues concerning our problem. However, just the mere possibility that the fault laid with me unsettled me beyond anything I'd expected — it was intolerable to live with. Why should she stay with me if I was the reason that she could not achieve her dream? I found myself being too critical towards myself, making it impossible to voice my concerns to Vas. I felt that if I voiced it, it would become true, and this terrified me.

Intellectually, I knew that firing blanks was a random illness (as I have repeatedly told my wife about infertility). Did that knowledge make it easier for me, to see it for what it was? No! I felt ashamed and started feeling less of a man. The feeling that I was not worthy of Vas and that she should not be with me, took root. I was angry at myself for firing blanks.

How stupid was that? However, it was still there. Logic went out of the window. I was actually feeling inferior to guys with children. Let me tell you; life had no meaning. What was the fucking point of my existence?

Vas's depression found a companion in mine. The only difference this time was that I was suffering behind a smile and a positive attitude. *I was the king!*

That was the second time in my life when what I was feeling and what I was projecting were two different things. I did not know at the time that, later on, I was going to develop that split persona into a finely crafted work of art.

It was the second time I'd indirectly lied to Vas.

You are probably thinking, "Come on, Steve. Stop being melodramatic. Stop seeking attention. A lie is when you actually say it aloud. You didn't tell your wife anything so, by default, you didn't lie."

The first step down the slippery slope is always one you can easily justify. Why did I get married? I wanted to share my life with my wife. Telling lies or not voicing what is troubling me falls well below the bar of sharing. Why get married to someone if you are going to cheat or lie to them? Save them the anguish.

But I needn't have worried — these lies were going to mean nothing compared to the massive lies I would tell Vas later on.

A long year later, I finally had the tests. Thankfully, my

swimmers came up trumps. Some of them were a bit lazy but, overall, they were functioning within normal parameters. I was virile. I was still the man!

The relief was unbelievable. No one could ever talk behind my back now. It was not my fault that Vas was not getting pregnant. The world made sense! I wanted to open a bottle of expensive malt whiskey and smoke a cigar. This was what my fear had reduced me to. It brought the short-sightedness and selfishness out in me.

Vas still had problems getting pregnant. As a couple, we were still facing the same problem. It made no difference to our lives that I was not firing blanks. Vas was still depressed, was still losing a bit of herself every day, and there was I relieved that I was not firing blanks. I was indeed ecstatic for a few days. Living with that fear had shaken me to the core, and I lost track of the whole picture. *I was the king!*

The good thing was that Vas was none the wiser. It may as well have been living with a stranger in so far as she knew what was going through my mind.

Well ...

Does this sound familiar to any of you? If it does, you have my sympathy, but not my understanding. If you are going through this torment as you are reading this book, do yourself a favor; talk to your wife. Tell her how you feel. Let her into your insecure world. Her reaction and support might surprise you! Don't do what I did. I thought I was strong when all I doing was showing weakness by not facing and sharing my fears.

What should I have done?

The moment I realized that I could have been firing blanks, I should have talked to my wife and gone to be checked out. If I were not firing blanks, then one problem would have been eliminated. If I were indeed firing blanks, then the doctors would have known, and I would have followed their advice and recommendations. If that were the case, I could have prevented Vas from tormenting herself — the fault would have been with me. Fear and pride prevented me from doing the right thing. I lived for a year with that fear hanging over my head. I was wrong. Unfortunately, I took that second step down the slippery slope.

The sooner you get checked, the better. Don't bury your head in the sand. The outcome will not change because you talked about it with your wife, but at least you'd be doing something constructive about it.

Worst case scenario, your fears materialize. Hopefully, it can be corrected. If not, you can consider donor sperm. I know it is not something you want to hear or consider, but at least it is available — you can still be a father. Irrespective of who the donor is, you will always be the father to that baby. The alternative may be living with the fear that your wife will eventually leave you. I have lived with that fear, and believe me, it eats you up inside. One way or the other, the earlier you deal with it, the better off you will be. There are always options as long as you have a compassionate and loving relationship with your wife. She will not leave you. She will fight tooth and nail to find a solution that works for the both of you.

At the very beginning when you decide to have a baby, donor sperm, surrogacy and adoption will never enter your mind. But now you are in no man's land and, unfortunately, you have to adapt. Communicate with your wife! How do you expect her to stand by you if she does not know what goes through your mind?

When Vas and I realized that we suffered from infertility, we both thought the problem was with her. By understanding her need to be a mother and by letting her know that you will be there for her even if the problem resides with her, you are being a good husband. If she finds that the problem is with you firing blanks, she will be there for you as well, for you deserve nothing less.

I read an article in the Daily Mail[13], relating to male fertility:

---

[13]http://www.dailymail.co.uk/femail/article-4776392/Silent-agony-husbands-haunted-male-infertility.html

It mentions a study highlighting that the sperm count of men in the Western world is declining. It also states that male fertility is falling off a cliff.

It is an issue that has to gain visibility in order to make men aware of the possible problems they might face. Support groups for men facing this challenge will be helpful as well. I found this problem devastating, but I was lucky as it wasn't real and only in my head. I dread to think how a man feels when he finds out he is firing blanks.

Some men might see firing blanks as a blow to their masculinity. Instead of looking at it for what it is, a random illness over which they have no control, they see it as a form of shame. They then suffer in silence, too embarrassed to talk about it as it makes them feel less of a man.

Going back to the four idiots:

Years later, I found that the first idiot was cheating on his wife. Needless to say, she left him. This is why I think it is better to avoid all the macho crap. Men who talk a lot about sex normally have problems with it. A friend of yours who tends to make fun of other people on a regular basis will eventually be making fun of you one day.

There is a saying in Cyprus: "Tell me who your friends are, and I'll tell you who you are."

I don't have many friends.

CHAPTER TEN

<u>DEALING WITH IVF</u>

"A couple's last chance saloon."

From my blog:www.vaspx.com

You have battled with infertility, month after month, for God knows how many years. The noblest of dreams still eludes you. You have hit the brick wall and finally admitted to yourself that you need help. Assistive Reproductive Technology is the only other option for infertile couples who still want to achieve their miracle. The most well known treatment is In Vitro Fertility (IVF). Of course, there is adoption and surrogacy.

What does IVF involve?

1. IVF can be a very expensive process.

2. There are no guarantees of success.

3. The woman's body is injected with chemicals, which cause hormone imbalances and may bring on the menopause earlier in her life.

4. Her eggs are then harvested, assuming she is capable of producing eggs.

5. The male ejaculates into a tube. The sperm is inserted into the eggs, which are then placed inside the woman.

6. The nail-biting waiting begins.

7. IVF is the last-chance saloon. If you cannot get pregnant with IVF, there is nothing else. This puts even more pressure on your glorious wife/partner.

8. I repeat: your wife/partner is the one who has to jump through all the hoops.

Simple, isn't it?

Except, there is a very thin line between success and failure.

The tough thing about IVF is that, should you fail at any part of the process, you cannot start the next IVF from where you failed the previous time. You start every single process from the beginning. A hurdle you successfully passed before might be the hurdle that fails during your current IVF attempt. On our first IVF, my wife successfully got pregnant. On the second IVF, the eggs did not fertilize. Same woman, same process, but the results were different. Let me tell you, it sucks! I shall go into the details later.

I am a man, and I found it overwhelming, even though my contribution was miniscule. My wife, like all women who undergo IVF, carried the burden all by herself, not once complaining, with total disregard for the possible long-term harm caused by the chemicals or the early arrival of menopause. Her health and safety never crossed her mind. She just wanted to be a mom. That is how deep her desire ran.

I read various articles on the internet claiming that, on average, a couple has to try at least six times before they are successful. Tell that to the poor souls who are on their eighth or tenth attempt. For those who are just about to start their sixth attempt, please, don't let this statistic raise your hopes — six is not a magic number.

Let us assume that every IVF attempt costs you $12,000 (including medication). If you take into account the days off work that you and your wife have to take throughout the process, the cost increases. A ballpark figure of $15,000 is not far off.

Scenario 1: You had six attempts and were successful on your last one. You are $90,000 in the red, but you have managed to achieve your miracle; your baby. You cannot put a price on life. Congrats!

Scenario 2: You had six attempts and still got no result. You are $90,000 in the red, with an emotionally scarred and devastated wife, and a life in limbo. She has battled with infertility, had six courses of IVF chemicals injected into her, and still no baby. That glorious woman needs your understanding, compassion, and love more than ever before.

Every time you have an unsuccessful IVF attempt, she will feel a failure. Her confidence and self-esteem will disappear. When men catch the 'flu,' our poor wives know all about it as we expect her to look after us. When my wife went through the IVF attempts, she never once complained. She had mood swings due to the chemicals, but she got on with it. Women are resilient and tough, but this infertility curse breaks them inside. Make sure you're there for her when she needs you.

You have faced infertility, and every month you faced the disappointment of the period raising its ugly head. You thought it was tough. Face IVF failure time after time, and the hopelessness you felt before becomes a happy memory.

You know that you have a budget as to how many IVF attempts you can undergo. Every time you fail … *more pressure.*

IVF is your last chance. If you cannot get pregnant with IVF … *more pressure.*

The chemicals that are injected in your wife …*more pressure.*

Nothing else matters in your life apart from having a baby. Everyone around you is getting pregnant … *more pressure.*

IVF can be devastating when you don't get a successful result. Many couples have split up after going through this harrowing experience.

Have you seen a boxer get punched so much his legs are like jelly, and he has a blank look on his face? How about a war veteran? The look of pain and fear on his face, full of anger ready to erupt! This is what I saw my wife deal with. This is how I think most women suffer when faced with infertility and one IVF failure after another. It was as if my wife had just come from a war. Defeated, scared, angry, and without hope. This is how bad it can get.

My wife embarked on IVF after living with the depression and frustration of infertility. To start with, she was hopeful as this was a new thing, but she was also scared as she contemplated failure. She could not help having these mixed feelings. Hope and fear! Reaching the end of the IVF process, where success and failure are out of your control, my wife was terrified. She just could not sleep. The day she was supposed to call the clinic to find out if she was pregnant, she was literary shaking with hope and fear. Getting told that she was not pregnant, she did look like the boxer and the war veteran. This is what women have to go through and the reason I go on about understanding and being there for them. These selfless and tortured souls deserve nothing less.

This is why I urge any couple considering IVF to have

an informed idea about both the positives and the negatives of this method. The actual outcome of the process will not change,but it will help them enormously should they face problems down the line.

When the going gets tough, remember:

- The likelihood is that it will not work the first few times.

- Be optimistic—know that, statistically speaking, it takes a few times. Should you fail, take it on the chin and soldier on.

- There is a bigger chance of birth defects for an IVF baby than one who is conceived naturally.

- There is a bigger chance of birth defects when you use a frozen embryo instead of a fresh one.

- After a few attempts, money will start getting tight. People might be tempted to look abroad to clinics who advertise IVF at a fraction of what they are paying back home. Would this result in similar outcomes as botched cosmetic surgeries?

- There's the danger of ovarian hyper stimulation—the woman's ovaries might balloon to the size of balls, putting her in mortal danger. It happened to us, and I almost lost my wife. Even though our GP knew she was undergoing IVF, he failed to reach the correct diagnosis. Had I checked how little he knew about it, we would have gotten in touch with the IVF clinic straight away.

Many things can go wrong. Having an informed idea about these things makes you stronger in facing them. It can also make you more likely to react quickly to problems. Our local doctor said that my wife had an infection and told her to drink plenty of water. If we knew about the possibility of ovarian hyper stimulation, we would have gotten in touch with the IVF clinic sooner instead of listening to our clueless doctor.

When we first attempted IVF, we were very optimistic. We faced a few problems, but we only knew the positives. We were not prepared. Ours was life and death.

I think we could have avoided a lot of panic and anger if we had a more detailed knowledge of the negatives.

Life has a way of throwing a spanner in the works. It is good to be in an optimistic state of mind but beware of naivety. Whether we are prepared or not, bad things can happen to us— being prepared is a way of prepared is a way of minimising the negative effects.

If nothing major happens, you have not lost anything by learning the possible negative outcomes. File them in your head and share them when someone you know goes through IVF.

If something negative happens, your knowledge and quick reaction might alter the outcome. If there is nothing you can do about it, at least it won't be such a terrible surprise — it will be tough, but you will hopefully cope better with your misfortune.

There can be complications in a normal pregnancy. Unfortunately, IVF brings its own complications. You might be desperate to have a baby, but don't treat IVF as a one-attempt obstacle. There are too many variables. Yes, you might get lucky, but to assume you will is naïve.

On the other hand, you should not lose heart should you learn that someone with the same infertility problems as you did not find success with IVF. It is different for every couple — my wife and a friend of ours both had polycystic ovaries. Both women with the same infertility problems went through IVF several years apart. Obviously, the other woman knew the terrible problems we'd gone through, and she was very worried that she could be facing the same fate. She went ahead with IVF and produced only one egg. It was not looking good.

Thankfully, she got pregnant, and everything went smoothly for her. She had her daughter. The following year, she got pregnant naturally, having another girl. Two women with the same condition faced different results through IVF. Don't compare yourself to other people. You are under enough pressure as it is.

I wish you all a safe journey in trying to achieve your miracle.

We suffered. We fought to achieve our miracle. We are VASPX.

CHAPTER ELEVEN

<u>IVF</u>

"Just dirty magazines and a bloody tube!"

We know women bear the IVF procedure all by themselves.

What you will read here is my account of what I saw of the process and of how my wife and I suffered at the time.

This is a couple's last-chance saloon.

When we first started to try to get pregnant, I thought that it was going to happen after a night of hot sex where I performed like a lion and the angels wept. That delusion disappeared quickly like mist in the morning.

Now expelled from my position as puppet, I now enrolled as a masturbator, as that was all that was required of me.

All I had to do was ejaculate into a tube. There were no angels weeping! There was no sex marathon! No congratulatory cigar! *I was the king!*

You might think it is nothing. I had to reach out and take the tube from a nurse, both of us knowing full well what I was going to be doing in a few minutes. My face was red. I did not look at her. I felt as if everyone was looking at me. I entered the room. I don't remember it exactly — there was probably a television and some porn videos. All I remember clearly are a few dirty magazines on a table. They looked worn. I dare not touch them for fear of catching something.

Knowing that everyone outside that room was waiting for me to do the deed made it more difficult for me to complete my task. Another thing playing on my mind was my swimmers missing the tube and ending up on the floor. I don't need to tell you that arousal did not come easily. I took ages, and it was a relief to see my swimmers finally in the tube. Surprisingly, they hardly filled the bottom. I expected it to overflow! Nevertheless, it felt momentous — I had finished my one and only function satisfactorily.

I still couldn't look at the nurse as I handed her the tube. We both knew what I had just done. When I went over to Vas and told her of my relief, she rolled her eyes. She never realized that since it was the only thing that I was supposed to do, my weird mind had been visualizing all the different ways it could have gone wrong. Irrespective of the rolling eyes and embarrassment, I felt proud of myself.

Another new job I acquired upon reaching the IVF stage was that of a punch bag. That's right — my wife's hormones were doing somersaults. I understood the pressure that she was going through.

Had the IVF failed as well, that would have been the end of the line for her dream. She felt scared as the cocktail of injections propelled her hormones to higher levels. She was right to react like that.

I knew all this intellectually, but did that knowledge make my new role any more bearable? Of course not. I am a man. Hormones are alien to me. When Vas kept quiet about feeling all over the place, I presumed she was her normal self. If I don't feel well, Vas knows all about it — when I finally shut up, it means that I am over it. I expected her to be the same. Therefore, when the next outburst materialized, it always caught me off guard.

What I am going to tell you next is a joke. It doesn't mean I don't understand women or that my views about women are outdated. If you are a woman reading the following joke, please don't let it stop you from reading the rest of the book. I know my jokes are bad. Apologies.

Women have a period every month for about half their lives. On one of Vas's (very rare) good days, I had a couple of beers (I tend to talk a lot when I have a drink), and the conversation turned to periods. I told her that after so many years of women having their period month after month, you'd think they would have learned to deal with it by now. They know it is coming, right? They have been experiencing the same pain month after month, year after year. Surely she should approach and deal with it as nothing more than a mild irritation!

All I got was an angry glare, and she stormed out of the living room. I ended up occupying the guest room for the night. Honestly, some people have no sense of humor; my superb, tasteful joke had been wasted. I had to remind myself to stop telling her any of my other jokes—sleeping in the guest room was rather lonely. *I was the king!*

The injections were a nightmare. First, they gave us the wrong needles, which made the first injection painful. After that, she could not help tensing up every time I readied the needle, which only made it more painful. She was screaming at me because my hand was not steady.

"Of course it's not bloody steady!" I'd tell her, shaking from the pressure, anticipating the screaming that I expected to follow.

My telling her, "Don't tense; otherwise, it will hurt," fell on deaf ears.

She kept yelling at me. "If you give me the injection nicely, there will be no need to tense!"

How can you argue with that kind of logic?

She was suffering, but so was I. Finally, we came to the last injection that had to go in her bum. The needle was massive. As soon as I saw it, I knew I was doomed. When it cut her skin, she started screaming. I had no wish to stop to comfort her. She would have screamed at me anyway. I was damned if I did, damned if I did not. I just pushed the needle in. I wanted the task to end. Vas is a very polite person with a very clean vocabulary — but that night it was X-rated. After it was all over, I tried to console her. She pushed me away in tears. Did she think that I'd done it on purpose?

Countless times during one of our blazing arguments (civilized on my part), the phone would ring, interrupting her yells. She then would transform into a paragon of calm — her voice would be tranquil, and she would laugh at their jokes. I'd think, "*How weird is this?*" When the phone call ended, she would once again transform into an angry beast, continuing the argument as if there had been no interruption. When I tackled her about being nice to her friends on the phone and shitty towards me, she explained that I was her husband. I was the only one with whom she could be shitty. Well, fair enough.

I reached the point that to deal with that time, I had to switch off altogether. We still loved each other, but Vas's scary hormones kept me on my toes.

I would sometimes catch her crying. I knew why. I would

just cuddle her and say nothing. What could I have said? "Don't worry, everything will be alright?" It was bad enough that others would tell her these empty and stupid words. Since there was nothing I could do to help her, I said nothing, but just was there for her.

All of the above happened from just one attempt of IVF. We had three. What joy!

Other couples have to go through many more attempts. I can only imagine the suffering and pain those couples go through, especially the women. God bless them.

If you look at IVF from a dispassionate and clinical perspective, you realize that it is just another form of lottery. You are playing the odds, hoping your numbers will come up. The fact that you have to overcome the various stages of the process before you get to achieve your goal makes it that much more difficult. I suppose this is why women's stress levels are way up there, for it is a daunting process. The depth of their desire, combined with the fear that it might not work, makes it a lethal cocktail for any man to live through. Well, it was for me. *I was the king!*

IVF is magical when it works. For us, it was indeed a miracle! Whoever has had a successful result with this method will praise it.

Those who only got misery and disappointment will condemn it.

However, it is the only method available when everything else fails.

The biggest disappointment with IVF for me was my miniscule contribution. In order to create my family, all I'd had to do was ejaculate into a tube.

"Come on! Ask me to climb to the top of a mountain and then ejaculate. I can live with that. Ask me to knock a wall down … just don't ask me merely to ejaculate into a tube. Don't take away my manhood." For such a critical event, I felt like an outsider.

No angels weeping! No two hours' sex marathon! No congratulatory cigar! Just dirty magazines and a bloody tube! *I was the king!*

Well …

The steps taken on any journey you embark upon with your wife will define how good a husband you are and how strong you will be when faced with problems along the way. Understanding the depth of your wife's need to be a mother while sharing your frustration about feeling like a puppet will enable your wife to understand you better and be more accepting when you sometimes tell her you are not in the mood during ovulation. Telling her that you will be there for her no matter what comes will create a greater bond. This will enable both of you to ride the storm.

If you had started like this, I can assure you that a stupid hang-up like ejaculating in a tube will never cross your mind. Both of you will face your battle as a unit, relying on communication, love, understanding, and compassion, and not allowing stupid and superficial feelings to disrupt the battle plan.

If this is all that is required from you, so be it. Instead of being resentful, be thankful, as this means that you have that much more time to be there for your wife, who will be doing everything else.

IVF might or might not work, but either way, you will not let it break you, for your marriage is made of sterner stuff. You will endure and fight the good fight because you must.

Can you see how a hypothetical scene is unfolding built upon the right steps? It stands in sharp contrast to my own real-life scene.

For every wrong step you take, you as a person change for the worse. I did!

Instead of appreciating my wife's personal hell and being supportive and understanding, I selfishly concentrated on stupid things. I was wrong. *I was the king!*

Another thing I found difficult to accept early on was all

the prodding in my wife's private area during egg collection. I wanted to grab the doctor by the throat. It was hard witnessing this scene, so I handled it by moving away and not looking at what was happening.

Three IVF attempts, however, knocked that out of me.

Our history:

I have to point out that all three IVF attempts took place within a short period of nine months.

On our first IVF attempt, out of twenty eggs, only one fertilised. The odds were against us, but we succeeded in getting pregnant. Vas was glowing.

Our second IVF attempt was a failure.

The third IVF was an experience I could have done without. Everything started going wrong within the first few days of Vas getting pregnant with twins.

Vas looked as if she was four months pregnant, within days into her pregnancy. As you know from the previous chapter, our local doctor thought it was a virus. As the pain got worse, Vas called the IVF clinic and had been told to urgently call an ambulance and that they would meet her at the hospital. She had ovarian hyper-stimulation, causing her ovaries to balloon to the size of balls. She was in excruciating pain, which placed her life as well as the babies in danger. I asked my mother-in-law to stay by the front door to let the ambulance crew in, while I remained with Vas. She was bent over clutching her belly and grunting in pain. The ambulance was taking forever.

My mother-in-law ran in all panicky, "Steve, the ambulance pulled up at the front of the house, but they sped off straight away. I raised my hands for them to come in the house, but the driver just smiled, cheerfully waved, and sped off."

My wife and the babies were in danger, and those bastards smiled and left. I am not a violent person, but I would have ended up in jail that day had I got my hands on them. I made a vow that had Vas or the twins died that day, I would have found out who they were and unknown to them, I would have paid them a visit.

Full of anger, I picked Vas up gently, put her in the car, and drove her to the hospital myself. They kept her in.

After three days, I brought her home.

Vas started taking folic acid as soon as she found out she was pregnant. After witnessing such a scary start, she also started a regime of mineral tablets[14] whose function is to improve your well-being.

When we went to 'Boots'[15], Vas took a small bottle of each mineral she wanted. I made a mental note of the ones she bought and the assistant who pointed us to the right aisle.

---

[14] See http://www.nordicnaturals.com/international.php and chapter 19

[15] See https://www.boots.com/

Once, she craved dark chocolate. I went to the nearest shop and I bought all they had. She went ballistic when she saw how many I got. This is why I went to Boots the next day without Vas knowing and sought out that assistant. I am quite memorable when I need help. I fumble my words, gesticulate (yes, I am Greek), and generally look lost and helpless, which I truly am. The assistant thought I looked like a puppy. I bought everything they had on the shelves. I wanted us to be well stocked. The other thing to understand, is by me taking this action, it gave me a purpose and something to do. My wife, like every other woman, was fighting this battle all by herself and I was just a spectator. I kept trying to find things to do much to Vas's annoyance.

Vas is a small built woman. She felt that her body had to be in tip top shape to withstand any possible problems. She was not wrong, was she?

Within three days, the pain would get unbearable again, and I would take her to hospital for a three-day stay.

That was not enough. She started bleeding and throwing up.

Pain, bleeding, and throwing up on an epic scale.

In the film *The Godfather*, there is a scene where a man wakes up, turns, and finds his bed bloodied and a horse's head lying next to him. This was our reality — my wife was right to scream, as she thought that she'd had a miscarriage. These scares wore on, night after night — waking up to those screams and that much blood breaks your confidence. Re-living this scene day after day obliterates hope. You become a nervous wreck and a defeatist.

Rushing her to hospital, I'd think the worst. The bleeding

would stop and then return, making its grand entrance at any time of the day or night. I lost track of the number of times I had to rush her to the hospital because she was either in pain, bleeding, or throwing up. Every single time was quite severe, placing the twins' lives in danger. As we drove to and from the hospital, my business began to fall apart as I was hardly there.

When she was puking, it looked as if a dam had burst open. There was no stop to it—I'd watch the life drain out of her and drop her off for three-day hospital visits. In the meantime, the pain from the ovarian hyper-stimulation was always there. She would come back from the hospital, and you could guarantee that within two or three days, I would be scared to near-death either from her screams if she was bleeding or her rushing to the toilet for that horrible throwing up. We got to know everyone at the hospital as Vas was spending more time there than at home.

I had to live through this recurring nightmare for the first four months of Vas's pregnancy.

We heard of a specialist in Harley Street, London. Our situation was dire, and we needed to get an independent opinion from someone who was an expert in that field. We wanted him to magically put everything right. We were that desperate! Since he was an expert, I thought we would find out one way or the other what our chances were to see this journey of ours through to the end.

We entered the clinic with worried frowns. The doctor's name was Professor Nicolaides. Never in my life have I met someone who so effortlessly put me at ease with his demeanor alone; he had a reassuring smile, and his voice was soft and yet oozed confidence and knowledge. I was hanging onto his every word. The stress and fear that had piled on top of me during the last few months were close to unbearable. Talking to Professor Nicolaides was like taking a breath of fresh air. He told us to try not to worry about it too much. The fact that Vas had fallen pregnant through IVF did not make it any different from any other pregnancy. We both felt rejuvenated after talking with him—I don't think we realized before how desperately we'd needed to hear some positive words.

It was not even that he did anything magical—he merely checked Vas and the babies and told us that so far, everything seemed to be okay. He took the time to explain in detail that what we were going through was not uncommon; it was a pregnancy after all. He could tell that we were worried to death. Apart from the ovarian hyper-stimulation, everything we were going through could have happened even if Vas had gotten pregnant the normal way.

I can still picture that meeting in my head. As he was talking, I felt myself become lighter as my pressures and worries were fought back. We'd just needed someone to talk to us in a friendly and compassionate manner. He was informative and not at all condescending—I came out knowing much more about pregnancy and IVF than when I'd gone in.

He stressed that we may still face problems. Unfortunately, anything can happen irrespective of how far gone a woman is. The only thing we could do was to try not to worry too much about it. He looked pointedly at me as he said those words! I guess my stupid questions gave me away.

When we left his clinic, there was a smile on our faces and a spring in our step.

We understood that we could still face problems, but we hoped that would not be the case—Professor Nicolaides would be our good luck charm.

Vas was four and a half months pregnant. With no hospital visits for a record of ten days (on Sunday), I took Vas to her parents, in Margate, for a break. She was glowing.

On Monday night, I received the first of three dreaded calls from my father-in-law. Vas had started bleeding heavily on the second day she was in Margate. He told me to stay and run the business since there was nothing I could do but stand and watch. Both my in-laws were with her. He would call me if it got worse.

On the phone to her every day, Vas and I would lie to

each other, pretending to have confidence that Vas would survive that scare. We had nothing to offer each other but these empty words of encouragement.

With no one to whom to vent my frustration and voice my fears, I again bottled it all inside. The vault of shitty feelings inside me was overflowing, ready to explode. I thought I could handle it. After all, it was my job to worry, not Vas's. Reaching out to anyone never crossed my mind, nor did I think I needed to.

The following weekend, I visited Vas. Her condition was as bad as I'd expected. It looked like total annihilation of our family. Vas was determined to do whatever was necessary to ensure that the babies survived. For her, it was make or break. She was at her own crossroads, petrified that history was going to repeat itself. The determined look on her face scared me. To what lengths would she be prepared to go in order to achieve her dream? Would I support her if it became critical? I didn't think so! Being in the middle of that battlefield, I made my mind up. This was going to be our very last chance. I had no wish to see Vas pregnant again if that meant there was even the slightest possibility of having to go through a similar ordeal. Of course, I didn't tell her this at the time. I hoped there would be no need.

On Monday, I returned home to try somehow keep my

business afloat. Every day and night, I thought about nothing apart from Vas and the babies. The helplessness was overwhelming—it was all out of my hands and so far away.

I was trying to be optimistic but was unable to keep in that frame of mind for more than ten seconds. What we had gone through had turned me into a defeatist—I'd honestly been a positive person before all of this happened.

Five days later, my father-in-law called the second time. Vas had started bleeding heavily and contracting at the same time. The hospital could not deal with babies so premature—she was only five months pregnant. They transferred her to Medway Maritime Hospital in Gillingham, about thirty miles away.

For those readers who have experienced a normal and uneventful pregnancy, try to remember how you felt when your wife/partner told you that her waters had broken. Full-scale panic at the beginning as you tried to remember to get everything and take the best possible route to the hospital. In the hospital, the panic is replaced by euphoria—you know your little miracle is about to make his/her grand entrance. With my wife at five months pregnant and carrying twins, there was no euphoria. The joke was on me!

Three long, agonizing hours later, the contractions stopped. We survived that scare, though Vas was still bleeding.

I went to see her that weekend. What I saw was the shell of the glorious and feisty woman I married. She was petrified. Since the contractions had made their presence known, I was sure they were going to grace us with another unwelcome visit. It was not unreasonable to assume this—it was us after all! Late on Sunday night, I returned home.

By Wednesday, the bleeding seemed to have slowed down, and we were cautiously optimistic. Maybe we were going to get the chance to see our journey to the end after all. The doctors told Vas they were thinking of discharging her at the end of the week. I was determined to bring her home where she belonged as soon as she stabilized.

My father-in-law made the third dreaded call on Friday evening. How I hated hearing his voice by then. It was always bad news! Vas was bleeding again; she was in danger, as were the twins. It had been two days since the doctors had told us they were going to discharge Vas, and now this—my worst nightmare come true. I got into my car and drove at dangerous speeds to the hospital. I honestly have no recollection of how I covered those two hundred miles —it's all a blur.

Unknown to me at the time, a few hours before, a nurse wheeled Vas to the operating theatre for an emergency caesarean. Vas was bleeding, but the blood was a dark color. Her years of experience kicked in and rightly concluded that Vas needed an emergency caesarean. However, the junior doctor in charge irresponsibly dismissed the experienced nurse's concerns, and Vas returned to her room. He felt it was not the nurse's place to make the call. Two hours after the incident, Vas started bleeding heavily, and this time there was no ambiguity about a caesarean. Total failure in due care. First, it was our clueless doctor, then the ambulance crew and now this junior doctor. When I found out about it, I made my second vow. He would have been the second person I visited. It felt as if obstacles and bungling professionals were placed in our path so that we could not achieve our dream. You cannot even begin to imagine the deranged hate I festered towards them.

I entered her room. My legs wobbled. She looked so weak. There was a bag of blood hanging beside her as doctors and nurses milled around her, performing blood transfusions and, at the same time, pulling blood clots out of her. She looked so scared! I tried to console her, but what could I say? I felt that I had to remain positive for her, even though I comforted her out of fear, panic, and desperation. It looked as if there was no hope for the twins and, to top that, Vas was in danger too. Worst of all was how Vas's desperation and yearning took over her common sense!

She voiced the unthinkable by wanting to refuse the caesarean. She hoped that with God's help, the twins would stay in her longer, giving them a better chance to come out alive.

Can you imagine your wife telling you such a thing when all you see around you are the imminent deaths of all the people you love?

It was all right for her to say that, but what about me? What about bloody me? As I said before, I'd been indifferent as to whether we had kids or not in the beginning. I married Vas because I loved her and because I wanted to spend the rest of my life with her. However, since I'd tasted that glorious feeling when Vas got pregnant with Xristos[16], everything changed. I wanted Vas *and* the babies in my life. I wanted to be a dad.

If I let Vas have her way, there would be nothing left for me. Absolutely nothing! No wife and no babies! She was willing to make me a widower on some delusion that her God would ensure that the twins survived if she placed herself in harm's way. My life was hanging on the edge of a cliff, hoping that an imaginary higher being would sort it out. Delusions!

If you have ever watched *The Deer Hunter*, you saw the scene with Christopher Walken playing Russian roulette with the loaded gun and the missing bullet. At least there was a bullet missing — the gun pointing at Vas's head was fully loaded. Once it fired, the only outcome was death.

Not even for a second could I let Vas entertain the idea that there was a chance I was going to agree.

---

[16] See chapter 11

The caesarean was to take place as soon as possible. I hated myself for shutting Vas down so absolutely since deep in my heart I knew that the babies would not make it. I did not want Vas to go to the operating theatre with her last memory of me being one where I'd been shitty to her. When I calmed down, I explained to her an edited version of my point of view. In between tears, she said she understood. I hoped she really did understand. We made our peace with each other and miserably waited for the trip to the operating theatre. We did not have to wait long.

As I was walking next to Vas, holding her hand as they whisked her to the operating theatre, she was crying uncontrollably. I reverted to stoicism, not wanting her to see that I was petrified.

Whoever said that men have to remain strong for their wives is wrong, and yet this is who I am.

Walking down that long corridor, expecting death to meet you as soon as that door opens, makes your legs tremble. You don't want that walk to continue, wishing you could go back into the room where you felt safe. You are scared, want to cry and scream because deep down in your heart you know that if you enter through that door, you will lose everything. You think you are screaming, asking them to stop, but not a sound leaves your mouth. The distance between you and that damned door keeps getting shorter.

Finally, the dreaded door opened.

CHAPTER TWELVE

ANGER AND ARGUMENTS

"None of you will have a bloody chance of surviving if you delay this. Do you hear me? None of you!"

The way I go through life is always in a committed, dedicated, and relentless way. Vas sometimes thinks I should be committed!

I got married. I decided early on that I would never get angry with my wife and never raise my voice to her. Whatever we go through, I feel I have to be strong for her. If I have to hide my feelings so that she knows she can lean on me, then so be it. If I cannot be there for her, then I have failed her. My views are a bit extreme, but this is who I am.

When Vas and I argue, I always want us to argue in a low tone and in a civilized manner. This winds her up even more, so she raises her voice to get a reaction from me. She says that since she is not a big woman; God gave her a big mouth to balance things. I think He overcompensated, but there you go!

A few years ago, we were at one of our neighbor's parties. I wanted to leave. When Vas did not want to leave, I suggested that she stay and I come back later. She knew I didn't intend to come back. I did not want to miss my favorite series, *Person of Interest*. This argument went on for about fifteen minutes. We talked in a low tone, and I had a smile on my face, which pissed her off even more. The other people around us thought that I was flirting with her, whispering sweet nothings in her ear. When Vas's friend told her this later, Vas rolled her eyes, informing her that actually we were having an argument. Her friend would not believe it.

This is how I always operated around her.

I was sometimes angry with her for being so fixated on trying to get pregnant. Seeing her sad because of her inability to do so prevented me from expressing my true feelings. I would have liked us to take a break sometimes to let a bit of laughter back into our lives. This was my failure to understand how deep her desire ran.

When Vas first refused to even entertain the idea of IVF, I was angry with her, but never voiced or showed my anger. She felt that by undergoing IVF, she was admitting failure. Come on! What difference would it make? Was it that important to get pregnant naturally? Surely, the end result is what counts. Because of Vas's stubbornness, I was still a puppet, and our lives were still in limbo.

Here's another example. Vas wanted to get a new car — a

Mini. Before I even had the chance to agree, she added the pre-condition that it had to be yellow with a black roof. For me, a Mini is a Mini. We ended up checking cars one-hundred-and-twenty miles away in order to find that particular color. I was not impressed. Okay, it looked good, but was it worth the hassle? If a car can get me from A to B, I don't particularly care what color it is. It was the same deal: whether Vas got pregnant the normal way or through IVF, it did not really matter to me. The important thing was to get a Mini or, in this case, a baby.

Should I have put my foot down, told her that enough was enough and to get on with the IVF? If I had known then what I know now, would I still have kept quiet? Of course, yes! There are certain things in our lives that I shall always follow Vas's lead.

When I did not voice my disagreement about her refusal to consider IVF, guess what, I failed her again. What is the point of looking strong for your wife when she does not have a clue what is going through your mind? If I had let Vas know my feelings about IVF, she might have reconsidered undergoing IVF instead of wasting a year. I was the instigator of most of my supposed 'suffering,' but I was too stupid to see it.

I was angry with cheerful people and suppliers. I had a supplier who was always very jolly in the morning. I told him a couple of times to just bring the delivery in and tell me how much it was without any cheerful chitchat. He was a reliable supplier, but the third time he came with his usual happy attitude (he dared to wish me good morning and actually asked me how I was that fine morning!), that really pissed me off. I sacked him there and then. What a jerk I was! He actually lost my business by being friendly. It was his bad luck that I was a monster. During that time, I sacked quite a few suppliers for no business-related reason whatsoever. I only kept the miserable and depressed ones who did not talk.

I was angry with myself for being useless at the time when my wife needed me the most. I knew it was out of my control, but that made no difference. I always prided myself on having a methodical and rational mind. It went out of the window together with everything else.

Most of all, I was angry with Vas when she wanted to risk her life when she was five-and-a-half months pregnant (on her third IVF attempt). That was the one and only time I spoke harshly to her. I have removed most of the swear words, for there were many:

Vas, "What can we do?"

"There is nothing we can do, Vas."

"It is too early for the twins to be born now. It is way too early."

"You have done well to carry them this far. You have done all you can do."

Vas's mothering instinct kicked in, and the shit hit the fan!

Vas: "I want to refuse the cesarean. This way, the twins will stay in me longer, and hopefully, this will help them survive."

I glared at my in-laws, and they hastily left the room.

The blood drained from my face. Was she out of her bloody mind? "If you think I am going to let you risk your life, you are wrong."

"Don't worry about me," she said. "With God's help, they will have a better chance of survival."

I could not fucking believe it. "Look at me!"

Vas refused to look at me.

"Damn it, look at me!"

She knew we were facing complete annihilation. She was in the middle of it, still clinging to religion and hope. All I saw around me was fucking death. My anger was beyond safe limits. My hands were shaking.

She finally looked at me.

"Are you out of your bloody mind?" I said. "You will die!"

I grabbed her hand and squeezed it hard. I stared at her

without blinking.

"Please!" Vas said. "It is their only chance."

"You will all die! All of you." I squeezed her hand even harder. I just could not believe what I was hearing. "Listen to me and listen well. There is no bloody way I am going to let you do this. You are having this cesarean as soon as possible."

"Please, Steve. It is their only chance!"

"None of you will have a bloody chance of surviving if you delay this. Do you hear me? None of you!"

"Please …"

"I don't want to bloody hear anything else from you."

Continuing to glare at her, my grip grew even harder. She had to understand that this was no debate. Even with a caesarean, there was no guarantee she or the twins were going to survive. She was completely white, as the blood transfusions could not keep up. All three of them had to take their chances. Any delay would have meant certain death for all of them. At least this way there was a chance for Vas, for I did not think the twins stood much chance.

On Wednesday, we were ecstatic when they told us they were thinking of discharging her because the bleeding had reduced drastically. On Friday, two lousy days later, they threw us into the cesspit of death again.

Vas never stopped to consider me. Had I agreed with her

decision, I would have been the only one walking out of that hospital, a beaten and broken man with only regrets, hate, and anger as companions.

In the end, Vas relented. She was in tears. I loosened my grip.

Even though this was within Vas's domain, I was certainly not going to follow her lead. How could I do that knowing that she would have died?

The utter terror I was living in at the time broke me. The fear of being left all alone, without a wife and babies, drove me near to madness.

When I calmed down, I tried to give her an edited version of my feelings. I did not want her to go under the knife with her last memory of me as someone cold and angry. We made our peace, getting ready to face the terror lurking in the operating theatre. We did not have to wait long. Little did we know, it was not just terror waiting for us. Death and madness were there to claim their bounty.

I hope none of you ever have to live through this kind of anger and helplessness.

CHAPTER THIRTEEN

<u>BIRTH</u>

**"How anyone can keep his sanity and humanity is beyond me,
for I lost mine."**

On our first IVF attempt, Vas got pregnant with Xristos. When
she was four months pregnant, an abnormality in her blood
ensured that more detailed tests were performed. To our shock,
Xristos was anencephalic[17]. He could not have possibly survived
had Vas gone full term. Vas was given a tablet to induce
pregnancy. She battled infertility for five years and got
pregnant. After coming so close, she had to give birth to our
angel knowing when he came out he would be dead. There is
just one word that can describe what I was feeling; Nothingness!

Our second experience with birth was on our third IVF
attempt when Vas was pregnant with twins. After our argument
about her wanting to refuse to have the caesarean, we entered
the operating theatre.

That argument unsettled me. It was not enough,

---

[17] See https://en.wikipedia.org/wiki/Anencephaly Absence of a major
portion of the brain, skull and scalp.

A doctor came over and asked me to sign some forms. As the twins were so premature, had they survived, they would then have to be on a ventilator. Apparently, there were two choices. The Conventional Ventilator (CV), and a new one called High-Frequency Oscillatory Ventilation (HFOV). He asked me to choose which ventilator to be given to which baby.

Unbelievable! A few hours before that, I was frying fish and chips. I then drove for two hundred miles like a lunatic. I had just spoken harshly to my wife for the first time ever, and this guy was asking me to choose. I had no idea about bloody ventilators. It hadn't even crossed my mind about the twins needing a ventilator.

The choice had to be made. What did I choose? I told him that the first baby out of Vas, to have the CV and the second to have the HFOV. Just like that, I decided their fate. A father ignorant about ventilators decided which baby was to have which ventilator. With dread and trembling hands, I signed the form. Did I just sign the deaths of my babies? Why did they make me choose? Would that decision come to haunt me later on? Damn you; damn you all and your carefree lives. *I was the king!*

I walked over to Vas. The caesarean was performed.

The first thing I remember was whilst standing there, I heard the consultant telling off one of the doctors (he was telling him off for delaying the caesarean), but I still did not understand their exchange as Vas had not informed me of the episode until days later.

The second thing I remember vividly was looking in my wife's inner body. If a sight like this does not bring you closer together, I don't know what does.

It was so surreal seeing the consultant put his hands in my wife's cut belly! Surrounded by so many professionals for those few seconds, I started feeling optimistic. It did not last long.

Andrea came out first and was handed to a doctor at the other end of the room. I followed. Her skin was dark, and I did not see any movement or hear a cry from her. Very quickly, he pronounced her dead. I went over and told Vas, who started crying. I could not afford to show any emotion. I had to be strong for her.

Inside my head, monsters were beckoning me to join them. I was sure they wouldn't have to wait long for my response, for if Petros died too, I would lose my wife. I would have not just joined them; I would have been the king of those monsters, for even they would have been scared of me.

Seeing my wife crying broke my heart. She looked so small and alone. The person that I was supposed to love and protect was in despair and heading quickly into the abyss.

And then they pulled Petros out.

He was the same dark color as Andrea. He wasn't moving or crying, and there, my life crumbled in front of me. It was a pathetic life over which I had no control.

The doctor tried to revive Petros for a few minutes. It felt like a lifetime. Finally, he stopped. "It's better if we let him die," he said.

"Please, keep trying."

"It's no use. It has been ten minutes."

He told me that since Petros had had no oxygen to his brain for ten minutes, even if he survived, he would most likely be brain dead. He was condemning me to a life with no babies, no wife, nothing. How the hell do you react to that? What actions do you take? Well, I was bloody dead inside. I just couldn't let him give up on Petros and, by default, my wife. How could I be expected to go back to her and tell her that Petros was dead as well? I couldn't deliver the news that would kill her inside forever.

The world was an evil place for me. I had experienced nothing but death and helplessness. I was just barely holding on to my own sanity.

Tears in my eyes, I told him, "If you stop, you aren't just killing my son, but also my wife. She will not be able to survive this. She will not be able to go home without at least one baby. Please, continue trying. Please!"

I begged him. My whole life was hanging in the balance, and which path it was going to take was in the hands of that stranger. Absolutely everything was out of my control. For me, those few seconds were going to define the course of my life—and they did.

All I could hear in my head, *"You are a failure as a husband! You are a failure as a father! You are a joke as a protector of your family!"*

They reduced me to nothing; you get to go through this pain, to have the privilege of having a glimpse of life without hope, dreams, laughter, and love. You get to know that you are actually standing outside the door of hell, begging it not to open. Deep in your heart, you know that as soon it does, your life as you know it is over.

Against his justified instincts, the doctor continued trying to revive Petros. He took pity on me, even though he told me that if by some miracle, the baby survived, he would be a vegetable.

After what seemed like hours, the doctor had Petros put in an incubator, and a nurse rushed him to the neo natal high dependency unit (NNHDU). That there still was no sign of life confused me even more. Was he dead or alive? What was happening?

The doctor walked quickly back to me and told me, "Don't get your hopes up, as he might not survive the trip to the unit."

Before I even finished nodding, he disappeared from the

operating theatre.

It was as if death was toying with me: "Don't get too comfortable. I am coming back. I am having a hell of a time messing with you."

I had to go back to my wife, who was going out of her mind. What could I tell her? The truth? Certainly not.

I could still see Andrea lying dead, forgotten as if she never existed or mattered.

That was my dead daughter lying there.

That was my barely alive son whisked away.

That was my wife waiting to fall into the abyss.

Do you see the irony of it all? Surrounded by so much death, physically I was the only one who was okay. How anyone can keep his sanity and humanity is beyond me, for I lost mine. Everything inside me became icy cold, including my heart. Love, hope, and compassion disseminated to nothing. Those were feelings that the rest of you kept and treasured in your carefree lives. Not mine. *I was the king!*

I found Vas gray-faced and worn. With a calm face and a shaky voice, I lied to her, telling her they had taken Petros to the NNHDU and that we would have to wait and see what would happen. No mention that he started the first ten minutes of his life with no heartbeat and no oxygen going to his brain, or the fact the doctor had told me that he might not even survive the trip to NNHDU. Right or wrong, by withholding things from

Vas, I felt I was protecting her. I hated myself for lying to her. *I was the king!*

Vas is the only person in whom I ever confided. However, with how she was feeling, I could not confide in her, as I thought she could not deal with the truth. I started being selective as to what part of the truth I felt she could handle and what parts she could not. For the time being, I was the only one who really knew that our lives were hanging by a thread. I was carrying the burden of knowing that Petros could have joined Xristos and Andrea any moment. Try living with that knowledge and that shame! One thing I can categorically say is that madness was not far off.

Our first visit to the NNHDU (soon after the caesarean), was utterly demoralizing. Petros had survived the first few hours, and was in the incubator, punctured by dozens of tubes and needles. He
weighed 685 grams; less than a bag of sugar. Vas broke down when she first saw him. He was so tiny, so unformed, and made no movements beyond what the ventilator did for him.

This is Petros's first picture.

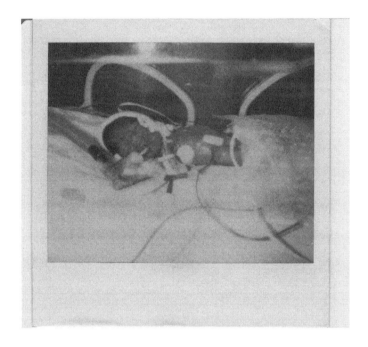

We couldn't see his eyes as his eyelids hadn't properly opened. He had no nipples! During those few minutes, the alarms went off constantly, and tireless nurses crowded around him, trying to stabilize him. Any hope I had that Petros was going to survive disappeared. I knew there and then that we were on a countdown to the total destruction of our family.

CHAPTER FOURTEEN

HATE
"It didn't matter what color, race, or sex. I hated every single one of you."

People deal with difficult times in their lives in different ways. I would like to think that most people keep their humane self. I, on the other hand, became an anti-social monster, full of hate. When I talk about hate, I mean pure hate. I nurtured it and helped it blossom. You see, in everything I do, I am committed, dedicated, and relentless. My hate was pure evil.

During Infertility Times

First, I hated myself. Getting someone pregnant is something that is easily achieved by most men. Not bloody me!

I hated the people who kept asking my wife if she was pregnant. I knew the result would be my wife crying for hours.

I hated the people who felt that they understood what my wife was going through. None of them had battled the monster of infertility, and yet there they were, dishing out understanding as if they were experts.

I hated the people calling to ask my wife if she'd had success yet. It is not the same as meeting up with someone and them asking you. You can choose not to go out and thus cut off any possibility of questions. Your home is your sanctuary. Once you close your front door, you can pull your hair, cry, bang your head on the wall, and feel sorry for yourself. Once you're home, no outsider can upset you. Our problem was that Vas's periods were quite irregular, ranging from twenty-eight to sixty days apart. During the long period cycles, they would call every single day.

How I hated those calls. Why couldn't Vas keep quiet? I never told my family, but word got to them through Vas's family, and they started calling as well. It was as if we were operating a call center. In the beginning, when the phone rang at home, I never bothered to answer it, as all my friends called me at the shop. I would then hear Vas say to whoever was calling, "No, not yet! I hope so …" They were actually telling her that they were sure she was going to get pregnant. I guess they had a crystal ball we did not know about. When the phone call ended, Vas would be in tears. I tried to console her while inwardly fuming.

In between sobs, she would say, "Why does it not happen for me …? What is wrong with me …? Why are you still with me …?"

Oh, how I wanted to inflict pain on the person who had just called! They felt they had done their good deed for the day, while my wife was sobbing her eyes out.

I called my parents and told them that whenever they called, never to ask Vas whether she was pregnant and never to tell her should any of our relatives have a baby. I told them to tell the same thing to the rest of our family. Immediately, my family's calls to the house reduced, with any conversation being safely pregnancy — and baby-free. It was a start.

"Have faith, and God will give you a child."

That used to get my back up. Vas is religious. Where was her God those five long years? Had He taken a sabbatical? Alternatively, were they implying that we were not spiritual enough for their God to grant that gift to us?

"Relax, don't think about it, and then you will get pregnant."

When you are living with this problem, you have enough crap to deal with. When people told my wife to relax and not to think about it, it brought violent feelings to the surface of my mind. My wife, like every other woman in this sad club, thought about nothing else. Rightly so!

Take my word for it. If you have an ounce of compassion and know anyone who is having trouble getting pregnant, never ask him or her about it. If they want to bring the subject up, fair enough. Never, ever ask them. You might feel you should reach out to show your support and worry that by not doing so you are being negligent in their hour of need, but better, more constructive ways exist for you to be there for your friend (see example at the end of the chapter).

Christenings were the worst. What is such a happy occasion for most people, for couples in our club, not so much! It is just another reminder of our failure. We are happy for the parents and their precious baby they brought into this world but don't wish to be reminded of our own misery.

For us, it went like this: when invited to a christening, Vas would go out to buy presents for the baby. When she came home, her eyes would be red. I never asked her why—what was the point? There she was, buying baby clothes for other people's babies instead of her own. I ended up trying to avoid situations where I thought we'd be invited to such events.

Everyone at these christenings felt it was their right to have a quiet word with Vas, telling her that they just knew she was going to have her own baby one day. No one felt comfortable approaching me, finding me a bit intimidating.

Trying to have a baby is not an illness where you can go to the doctor, get some antibiotics, and then get better within a few days. It is not an operation after which you can make a full recovery. If you are having problems getting pregnant, it can sometimes take years to achieve your dream. Sometimes, sadly, it never happens. Good wishes and keeping your fingers crossed aren't going to do anything for these tortured souls.

In the beginning when people kept asking us if there were any kids on the horizon, I did not mind their questions.

I even thought my response ("We are practicing!") was quite witty.

However, time took its toll. When were we going to see a result? How long would I have to keep seeing my wife sad and depressed?

With everyone around us getting pregnant, why the hell was it not happening for us? These were the frustrating questions circling around my head. I never talked about it with Vas. I did not know how!

Vas thought I was unaffected by the experience. She was wrong. I suffered, the same way as any other husband does, in silence. This is where I failed my wife. I failed to appreciate the depth of her need. When she was venting that frustration, I dared to think that I was unjustly suffering. *I was the king!*

Most of this hate could have been avoided had we not shared our plan of trying to get pregnant.

My failure as a good human being did not end there. It blossomed!

1st IVF attempt

My descent to monster started when we lost Xristos. He was anencephalic. I knew we were not the only ones who had who had suffered a loss like this, but I could not care less about the others. *I was the king!*

I just could not come to terms with it. The injustice and cruelty of fate.

Where we were planning how to decorate the nursery, we were putting him in a coffin. Instead of guiding and nurturing him, we were burying him. I was picturing the house echoing from his laughter; all I could hear was Vas's screams.

"Don't bloody tell me that you understand and to have faith. You have no idea what I am going through. I don't care to hear what you want to say." *I was the king!*

2nd IVF Attempt

…Failure

I hated pregnant couples. Why could they get pregnant so easily when we went for years without any success? *I was the king!*

3rd IVF Attempt

I hated myself for breathing when my first two babies had died without taking their first breath. I hated myself for being able to breathe, while Petros could not breathe on his own. I hated myself for being a picture of health while my wife was dying in another hospital. I stopped looking in the mirror. Whether I was shaving or combing my hair, it was done in a hurry. Every time I looked at myself in the mirror, it was with disgust, hate, and anger.

My in-laws and I get on just great, but during the IVF and early birth, I was horrible to them. There was no reason or justification. I think it was because, despite all my mistakes, they were still nice to me. I did not just get a great wife when I married wisely—I got great in-laws.

I started hating them as well. What had they done? They dared to ask me if I needed anything. They had the nerve to ask if I could go to their house to eat a cooked meal instead of living on pizzas and burgers. They dared to bring me food, which I refused to eat. They had the audacity to be concerned about their daughter and grandson. They dared to panic when it looked like their daughter and grandson were going to die. When you reach the stage I reached, logic goes out of the window.

They were the ones who had given birth to Vas and raised her. She had spent most of her life with them. In the blink of an eye, I considered them outsiders. Their daughter was dying, and I shut them out. My mother–in-law panics easily—that is her nature. Her way of coping with the potential annihilation was to go to NNHDU to see Petros and ask the nurses how he was progressing. Now, you have to realize, those nurses had to be on the ball, always available to respond at a moment's notice. When a baby needed their help, any delay could have meant death for that baby. Vas had only seen Petros once. I kept going to report back to her. On the third day, a nurse asked to talk to me. She said that my mother-in-law and the rest of

Vas's family were actually taking up a lot of their time with their frequent visits. It only took me a fraction of a second to decide on a response.

"From now on, no one is allowed to see Petros apart from Vas and myself."

With those few words, I denied access to everybody. That could have meant the difference between life and death as far as Petros was concerned. Other people's feelings were irrelevant to me. My mother-in-law was spitting feathers. My father-in-law approached me and asked me to reconsider.

"Steve, please, let Anne see Petros. She is going out of her mind with worry."

Very sharply, to my shame, I told him, "I shall allow no one to take up any more of the nurses' time."

There was no debate. I was done talking. Instead of having a civilized conversation and asking them to reduce their visits, I cut them all out. In my eyes, I was the only one suffering, and I hated them for intruding in my miserable life. *I was the king!*

There were moments when I found myself trembling. I wondered if Iwas going crazy. I didn't consider that others could have been suffering as well. I couldn't care less about anyone else's feelings. *I was the king!*

I hated parents whose babies were in the same unit as Petros. They had the nerve to try to talk to me. They wanted to give and get support from people in the same club. They had the same worries as me. However, whichever hospital I left, death was hovering around my family. It was bad enough enduring the quiet chats with the consultant. All it took was a deranged glare, and they would retreat, never to try again. I would see them whispering whenever I went past, which did not bother me in the slightest. They were not worthy of joining my club. *I was the king!*

I hated people leaving the hospital with their newborn babies in their arms, all smiles and happiness. Their babies had been admitted weeks or days after Petros had taken root there. Where was the justice in that? Why could I not taste that sort of happiness? Why could it not be them stuck in the hospital, worrying every day about when their kin would die, while I left the hospital with my wife and my baby? *I was the king!*

I hated you! Yes, you. I didn't know you, but thinking you could have possibly lived a happy and carefree life made hate you, for I was no longer one of you. I was politically correct; it didn't matter what color, race, or sex you were. I hated every single one of you. *I was the king!*

I hated priests; charlatans just selling a myth.

I hated God. I knew He didn't exist, that religion was a method of controlling the masses. On the off-chance that I was wrong, I made sure to hate Him with a passion. I think I hated

Him the most—how could he be just and loving? I hated Him because my wife had been willing to sacrifice her life in her wrong belief that He existed. *I was the king!*

There was no need for anyone to try to scare a kid with the bogeyman. Threatening any kid with the prospect of my presence would have made them toe the line, for I was scarier than any imaginary monster.

When you reach this level of pure and concentrated hate, there is nothing good inside you. Your very being becomes a black mass and, by default, you become evil. I projected that kind of evil wherever I went, for that was what I was. I felt alone, scared, and to mask the fear, I immersed myself in hate. It kept me sane. *I was the king!*

Well ...

If I try to fully analyze the extent of my hate and pinpoint where I went wrong, I may burden you with another book. I shall not do that.

My hate was pure and evil. I suppose I held on to it to stop myself from having to deal with my fears, shortcomings, despair, selfishness, and stupidity.

Even as I am writing this book, I can still taste the hate in my mouth. It has been eighteen years, but it was in such a pure form, so vile and evil, that to my shame I can still feel it. I was basking in it every day. It was unwarranted, unreasonable, and illogical. The well was bottomless. At the time, I thought I was right to hate everyone. For this, I am ashamed and remorseful. Reliving this feeling brought to the surface just how lost I was. I felt there was no way back for me, for I was evil. These are not just words.

By not taking that first wrong step, I could have avoided slipping into such hatred — but I took it anyway. What does that say about me?

What steps you take will determine the path your life will take. If it is not a good one, just blame yourself. Don't take your anger out on others.

I have been there. Through the grace of God, I got lucky in the end. Had I not, I would have had no chance to rebuild my life.

I can't stress this enough. Please, don't make the mistakes I made.

***

Someone I know was going through the same problem of infertility. I always treated him as if everything was normal in his life. We met at a wedding, and I asked him if I could have a quiet word.

When we were alone, I told him this:

"I am going to tell you something. I don't want you to interrupt me. After I finish, I still don't want you to tell me anything about what I told you. Are we in agreement?"

I don't have many friends. The few that I have know very well when I am serious. If I ask them for something, I shall not accept any deviation from our agreement. He nodded, more curious than anything else.

"I know what you are going through. You know that I have been through the same. I shall never intrude in your life. Know this; if ever you are feeling down, and you want to talk, I am here for you. Come and see me at the shop or call. Any time! Now I've finished what I wanted to tell you. By the way, it is your round."

He looked at me, and for a split second, I could see the pain in his eyes. He tried to talk, and I shook my head, not allowing him to speak. He kept looking at me.

"Stop looking at me like that. This isn't our wedding!"

He burst out laughing. I grabbed him by the shoulder, leading him to the bar. He still had to pay for the drinks! I told him about a guy I knew who had bragged that he had to stand on a stool to pee because his penis was that long. More laughter ensued. He'd come here to escape. I would be damned if I was going to take him back to his hell. Before we left, he looked at me, nodding his head.

What do you think? Was this a better way of reaching out

to him?

Do you think that just blurting, "Any news? Is your wife pregnant?" would have been better? I think that, by asking this direct question, I'd have been forcing an answer from my friend irrespective of whether he wanted to talk about it or not. I knew his pain was that great—I wanted him to know that he should talk about it only when he wanted.

We each have our own way of approaching delicate subjects with friends. Think long and hard to find the least painful way to be there for them. When he/she is ready to talk, just listen. Always looking him/her in the eye.

*Don't say that you understand.
Your friend doesn't want/need to hear this. Unless you've lived through this yourself, you don't understand and you won't in a million years.

*Don't blurt things out of ignorance.
Relax and it will happen for you. You are young and you have plenty of time. Is it your fault you aren't getting pregnant or your husband's?

*Don't suggest IVF, surrogacy or adoption.
It isn't for you to find a solution for them. If anyone is going to decide this, it is your friend and only when he/she comes to terms with it.

*Just listen. This is the best gift you can offer.

When the conversation ends, for God's sake, don't pick up the phone to share it with your best friend, mother, brother, or sister. The information is not yours to share—it is the private and personal suffering of a tortured soul. Treat it with the respect it deserves. Otherwise, you were never the right person to confide to in the first place.

CHAPTER FIFTEEN

<u>FAITH</u>

"If her God existed, where was He when we needed Him the most? Did He decide to have a day off?"

Some people are religious, and some are not. It is everyone's right to choose whether to believe or not.

I am a Christian Orthodox. I wasn't particularly bothered by or interested in religion and have always kept away from discussions or debates about it. It just wasn't my cup of tea. I guess you could have called me an "Indifferent Christian." That said, I still went to church with Vas as it was important to her. Because they have to cover so much during the service, they would up the tempo on the hymns, meaning I could never understand a single word. Most of the time, I would go over the list of the things I had to do the following day or else would listen to a whispered conversation going on nearby. I'd almost certainly be very bored and would drift off, thinking of a dozen other places I could be.

But what can God do for members of our unhappy club? Well, religious people will tell you that you should pray, for God will answer your prayers. Idiots! We've already been to church. We've been praying for years. I understand Him not answering *my* prayers, but my wife is quite devout. *I was the king!*

You see strangers walking around with babies or bumps in their bellies. Where is the justice in that? If there was a just God, why did He not throw a bit of justice our way? Why did we still have to suffer? *I was the king!*

As you know during our first IVF treatment, Vas got pregnant. We decided to call him Xristos (after Jesus Christ). He was going to be our miracle baby. Even an 'Indifferent Christian' like me thought it was appropriate. Of course he was born dead.

This was when religion, even if I had flirted with it for a while, went out of the window. Vas was shattered and inconsolable. Stupid people would approach me, feeling that they had to give me their support and impart their wisdom.

"Have faith, I'm sure your baby is with God," they would say.

Idiots! My baby should be with me and certainly not with their God. All I wanted to tell them and their imaginary God was to get lost and piss off out of my life. I did that many times. *I was the king!*

How delusional could they have been?

Priests came to comfort me. Of course, they were just trying to sell me their religion.

"Where was He when my baby died?" I said. "Where were His benevolence and love? Why did He not help Xristos join us in this world alive? Don't come preaching to me that my baby is up there with Him. Don't come preaching to me that it was because it was my son's time to meet his maker. There is just one word for all this: bullshit!"

To those who did not get the message and instantly retreat, I said: "Stand in the cemetery while they are lowering my baby's coffin into the grave and then tell me to have faith and believe in God. Make sure you wear body armor and take out life insurance! I don't need your comfort. I don't need your support. I don't care what you have to say. I need my baby. Can you bring my baby back to me? Of course not! Unless you can do something to bring my baby back to me, shut up, and keep your distance. Now is not the time for talking!" *I was the king!*

Have you ever encountered a Greek-Cypriot wishing to support you with religion in your hour of need? Unfortunately, I have. They get emotional and are in your face. Where one word would suffice, they will use ten. They will not stop until they feel they have exhausted all they have to say. It doesn't end there; they will hang around just in case they get any last-minute inspiration, which they will then insist on dumping on you.

Many of them were the same people who had upset my wife by asking her if she was pregnant. If they hadn't had problems getting pregnant, they knew someone who had. If they hadn't lost a baby, they knew someone who had. If they weren't having a bad hair day, they knew someone who was. They were relentless. You may think I talk a lot now, but back in the day, I was not much of a talker. I was (and still am) more of a listener. However, I didn't want to listen to their crappy stories about the butcher of the cousin of a friend of theirs who lost a relative fifteen years ago. I did not care about the butcher, the cousin, their friend, or them. As a group, they could all take a flying jump as far as I was concerned. *I was the king!*

I spoke to one man who had lost his teenage son a couple of years back. He told me how a mutual acquaintance had approached him in the cemetery on the day he'd buried his son. That guy had actually told him about losing a member of his family ten years before and told the grieving father to have faith. Apparently, it took the man forever to finish the story—he wanted to show him that he knew how he felt. That man had just buried his son—he didn't care whether the other person knew or didn't know how he felt. He was crushed! He told me that, for a split-second, he had wanted to laugh at the absurdity of that person's idiocy.

After we lost Xristos, others felt that they had to tell me that they knew what I was going through as well. Why did they feel the need to do that? Had they lost a child or were members of their family close to dying? If not, then they couldn't have known even in their wildest nightmares what I was going through. If they had lived through something similar, then they should have remembered how they must have felt at the time. They should have known that silence is the greatest thing you can offer someone grieving. Unfortunately, Greek-Cypriots and silence don't go together. We as a people love to gesticulate. How I wanted to chop those fucking hands off! They tried to ram religion down my throat because that was what made sense to them. In their cocoon, "God's will" allowed them to get through anything. Look at history—look at the number of gods for whom men, women, and children have been killed. How are today's gods any different? Same stupid people, same bullshit— just different names for the trending gods. *I was the king!*

These were the angry thoughts that were going through my mind: *Life just had no meaning. What was the point of it all? One word kept popping into my mind: nothingness. Life, our whole fucking existence, counted for nothing.*

I hit rock bottom. Well, I thought I did.

During our third IVF treatment, my wife finally got pregnant with twins!

She was prepared to turn me into a widower based on some deluded belief that her God existed. I would have been turning in my grave a thousand years from now when it is finally established that He never existed in the first place. Do you remember the Greeks and their gods on Mount Olympus? They were devoted to their imaginary gods, just as I felt that my wife was falsely devoted to hers. *I was the king!*

One of the twins died, and the other one and my wife were left fighting for their lives.

Here is where I realized that, if there was a hell, I was living in it.

Life could not get any worse, or so I thought.

If her God existed, where was He when we needed Him most? Was He having a day off?

I had been indifferent to religion before, but now it all changed. I knew! I definitely knew that there was no God. The only person I allowed to continue talking to me about God and faith was my mother. She called me from Cyprus, beside herself with worry, telling me to have faith and to never to give up. I was tolerant just because she is my mother, but sometimes, when I couldn't bear to hear any more of it, I would cut the conversation short. It was a pleasure to talk with my dad—he was a man of a few words. *I was the king!*

Facing this kind of sorrow propels you to such lows that

love and compassion become alien to you.

When you meet someone who is suffering or has just undergone a loss like this, the only possible humane thing you can do, according to me, is to nod your head and say nothing. Keep your mouth shut—what that person is going through at that time has no cure. He does not want to talk, and he is in no fit state to listen to your stupid words of encouragement or faith. *I was the king!*

Sometimes, silence speaks volumes. So much talking when all you need is quiet.

When I was ill, it was the only time I didn't want Vas to talk to me, and I especially resented questions that required an answer from me. If I was like that with Vas, how could I be expected to tolerate anyone else? I was about to lose everything that gave meaning to my life.

You might be thinking that I was unreasonable to expect people to react to my way of thinking. Wherever I am, I always try to suss out who I am in the company of, whether they like or don't like to talk a lot, if they can take a joke, etc. I always try to make sure that what comes out of my mouth doesn't cause distress to others. I expect nothing less from people who are in my company. I never got that kind of empathy from anyone. I only needed someone to sit next to me without uttering a single word. I never got it. Instead, all I got were the words of a righteous God whom I wanted to tell to take a flying jump.

With nothing to believe in and with my family's existence on a countdown, I was left all alone with my hatred. Welcome to my kingdom, for *I was the king!*

Soon after Vas gave birth to Petros, her body shut down. Three weeks later, as Vas looked like she was close to dying, my mother-in-law suggested bringing in her priest so that Vas could have Holy Communion and a blessing. I totally blanked her. My silence, as far as I was concerned, was an emphatic "No" to her request. She knew my views on religion. I'd had a shitty day that day, having just done the sixty miles round trip after visiting Petros. He was having one of his touch-and-go days.

Enduring that scene with Petros, the obligatory chat with the consultant, and seeing my wife on her not-far-off date with death was just too much. Bloody religion and its delusional followers. Why could they not accept that there was no heaven? Why did they not realize that the life they were living was the actual hell their Bible described? Why could they not believe and practice their delusions in the privacy of their own homes, without raising my anger to dangerous levels? I was living in the cesspit of death, and Vas's mother had the nerve to mention religion in my presence. If Vas hadn't been there, I would have exploded. Absolutely everyone was outside our bubble. *I was the king!*

Reaching that stage of idiocy and evil is not something one achieves easily. To start with, you must already have it in you. I had oceans of it.

The following day, I was in Vas's room. The curtains were shut tight, and the lights were out. Complete darkness. The hope was that Vas would get some much-needed sleep. I was sitting at her bedside, drowning in my misery. I heard loud voices outside the room. I ignored them. A few seconds later, the door suddenly swung open, and a tall, dark menacing figure entered the room with something swishing around him. I honestly thought he was Grim Reaper coming to claim his bounty. I jumped out of my skin. Not a sound came from him. For a grown man to be that scared, to honestly believe that the Grim Reaper was about to claim his wife, shows you a glimpse of my headspace.

The lights were suddenly turned on. To my relief and anger, I saw the local priest. Greek priests always dress in loose, swishing black clothes and wear long beards and tall black caps on their heads. My mother-in-law had defied me. When I'd overcome my initial terror, I threw her a dirty look that she totally ignored. Her daughter was dying, and she was in pain, but I couldn't see that.

What did the blessing and the Holy Communion

achieve? Nothing! On the contrary, they inflicted more pain on Vas. We woke her from sleep, which by then she could only achieve through sheer exhaustion or drugs. I am sure that Vas didn't understand a single word the priest was saying, as these charlatans use the old Greek. I guess they feel that they have to provide some kind of mystic atmosphere to make the crap they are selling more appealing. I was not a sheep, and I was certainly not buying into his bullshit. I was the king!

Well ...

I felt I was unjustly suffering. I blamed my misfortune on an evil God. My view was that, as my life was not full of roses, there was no God. Talk about selfish, narrow-minded, and stupid.

The trials we face test our mettle and character. In complete denial, to hide my weak nature, I focused on a God who wasn't righteous and loving. Concentrating on that enabled me not to deal with my shortcomings. *I was the king!*

I never considered that everything had started with my first lie and first wrong step. We all suffer one way or the other. Some trials we go through may seem to us to be extreme.

What I should have done was accept our situation for what it was and realize that the world did not revolve around me. I should have given support to people in the same boat as me and allowed help from friends and family. Faith would not have been far off.

Vas returned to her room soon after we saw Petros for the very first time. A few hours later her body shut down. She could not eat or drink. The doctors were baffled. The only explanation they could come up with was post-natal depression. It affects a lot of women. I am not a doctor, so I accepted what they said. However, her symptoms included an alarming loss of weight, constant pain, and non-stop throwing up. Within a couple of days, she was thinner than she had been before she'd got pregnant. It didn't make sense. Vas was insistent that their diagnosis was wrong; her statement was enough for me.

I had a meeting with the consultant, which proved to be useless. He claimed there was nothing else they could do for her as she was in denial. They stubbornly stuck to that diagnosis as nothing else made sense to them. I wanted to take Vas to a private hospital in London for a second opinion. They threatened me, saying that once we left, they would not re-admit her. I'd had just about enough. I was on the warpath. My first action was to call the chief executive's office. I told his secretary of my grievances and threatened them with litigation. My complaint was on record now. As if by magic, a new team of doctors met with me.

My father-in-law wanted to be at the meeting.

Let me tell you some things about my father-in-law: during the first years of marrying Vas, whenever I called him for a chat, I would say, "Hi, Andrew. Are you okay?"

Andrew would say, "Hi, son. Yes, thank you, and you? How many times have I asked you to call me Dad?"

I would laugh and totally ignore his request.

During our tough times, whenever I called him, it would be with bad news. "Andrew, Vas is bleeding. Can you come up, please?"

"Of course, son," he would say. "I shall see you in five hours." (He is a slow driver!)

He had his own business and, whenever I called him, he would literary drop everything and come up. We were very close, even though I never called him "Dad" and continuously teased him about his political beliefs. Great in-laws!

As soon as we entered the room, my father-in-law went about shaking everyone's hand. He then said, "Hello everybody. Thank you for taking the time to see us today. I hope you are all keeping well."

One of the doctors said, "It is our pleasure. We hope you are both keeping well too."

Unbelievable! My wife was dying, and they were exchanging pleasantries! For all I knew, she could have taken her last breath during those stupid pleasantries. We all knew why we were there. My complaint was on record.

I grabbed my father-in-law's hand and hissed harshly in his ear, "Please, stop."

I took point at the meeting, and in a loud voice, I expressed my grievances. They asked me to calm down. How could I? Words like: "negligence,""incompetence," and "litigation" were flying out of my mouth. I was threatening, insulting, and alienating the very people that I wanted to save my wife. *I was the king!*

When I was angry or in any way stressed, I had a habit of switching from English to Greek in between sentences. That was the first time I didn't do that.

Vas was dying, and Andrew was still polite to people. Even though he knew I was wrong in the way I was talking to them, he never said a word; just because I'd asked him to stop talking. He did that not because he was afraid of me, but because he knew I was better than that and was hoping I would find my way back to my old self. Bless him!

A barrage of new tests was scheduled and carried out. One of the tests was conducted by the consultant who was caring for Vas at the time. I think he was still angry with my complaint and took it out on Vas. He carried out a procedure and, where he should have used an anesthetic, he didn't. Vas was in tears. My wife was dying, and he had the nerve to inflict pain on her.

I did not tell Vas that I was the cause of that rough procedure because of how I'd treated them at the meeting. *I was the king!*

That doctor would have been the third person I visited. I don't know why, but I never included the very first doctor who failed to diagnose the ovarian hyper-stimulation. I was so scared and petrified and in order to cope with my fear of being left alone, I tried to fill the future emptiness with these visits. I was in a bad place. You might think that that was an empty threat. Remember this: I am committed, dedicated, and relentless. On a dark, cold, and rainy night, I would have paid them a visit. The problem was that the bloody list kept growing.

When the incident with the ambulance crew happened, I wrote a letter to the Chief Executive of the Ambulance service, expressing my disgust and threatened him with litigation. I got in touch with my lawyers and got ready for battle. I told Vas about my intentions.

"Please let it go."

"Vas, someone has to pay for this."

"Listen to me. The babies are okay as well as me. We don't need this hassle."

"The guy from the ambulance service asked me to name a convenient place, so we can meet and resolve the matter amicably."

"Why don't you do that then?"

"I can't. He'll probably say something 'amicable', and I just know I shall grab him by the collar and end up beating the crap out of him."

"I know you. You are like a dog with a bone. Ten years down the line, and you will still haunt that poor man. Please, let it go."

Much to my disagreement, I let it go just because she asked me. With Vas dead, there would have been no one to stop the pain I intended to inflict. I was deranged, and at the same time, I was the king!

I found my reality depressing, scary, and overwhelming. Whenever I closed my eyes, I retreated to my hell. Just nothingness! No wife and no babies. It was dark and cold, and in the far distance, I could see piercing bright red eyes and hear the screams coming from those monsters. Eyes open or shut did not make a fucking difference. My life sucked. My way of coping was by creating an isolated world in the farthest corner of my hell.

Since it was my world, I was all mighty and powerful. This is the surprise. For an unsociable person, I made sure I had guests. They were the ambulance crew and the two doctors (so far!).

They were all tied to a chair, and their mouths were shut tight because even in this world I did not want anyone talking to me.

With a voice like thunder I yelled at them, "I hold you

responsible for the deaths of my wife and babies. What have you got to say for yourselves?"

They squirmed, and I could see the muscles of their mouths move, but not a sound escaped.

In a low whisper as if I was talking to a lover, I asked them. "Why did you let my wife and babies die?" It was low and soft but full of venom. They struggled to hear me. I could see their confusion. Was I still angry?

It did not last long. They looked into my eyes seeking confirmation that they were safe. The eyes are the gates to the soul. They don't lie. When they looked into my eyes, they trembled, and beads of sweat rolled down their foreheads. What else did they expect to see in the eyes of a monster? I could taste their fear for they sensed what was coming.

I sometimes had them in a boxing ring with teeth and blood flying everywhere. Other times, I used my fish knife. In every case, I could sense their screams wanting to come out of their mouths, but only their tears ran freely. Their eyes were a treasure. They bulged out in disbelief, and then they shrank in terror. I was not going anywhere. I had nowhere to go. I intended to punish, and punish I did. The only thing that would stop me was remorse. When I saw it in their eyes, I sometimes grabbed their noses or held their heads in my huge hands and … This last scene was the trigger that enabled me to open my eyes and face the present.

Do you want to hear something disturbing? I found it soothing being there. Knowing that the pain, blood, and terror were experienced by someone other than me was exhilarating. Revenge is a dish best served cold. Never mind cold, mine was icy and deadly. Every time I rejoined my reality, I felt a bit better. I guess this was why I spent so much time there. The sad thing was–that fantasy had a good chance of becoming a reality.

There is a thin line between sanity and madness. In complete denial, I was tilting into madness thinking that the only suffering I was experiencing was a tiny bit of anger and hate. The problem was that I was turning into a dangerous madman. I was the king!

Instead of holding someone accountable for my loss, I should have smashed things, screamed, cried, and mourned. I should have dealt with my bloody emotions. That would have prevented me from sinking so low and becoming a potential murderous psychopath. All this ugliness, from a dream of becoming a dad.

The doctors were still bloody baffled. Nothing showed up that could explain Vas's body collapsing. She was throwing up green bile thirty to forty times a day and hadn't eaten or drunk anything for three whole weeks. They had to give her nutrients intravenously through a drip.

We were expecting her to die at any moment. Just looking at her, I couldn't tell whether she was alive or dead.

Soon after the priest who scared me, performed his religious 'voodoo,' he and my in-laws left—it was evident from my demeanor that I didn't want them there. Vas told me that as soon as she'd drank the Holy Communion, she'd felt as if hot hands were spreading and touching every inch of her body. I thought she was hallucinating and just nodded.

Here comes the kicker! Two hours later, she told me that whatever had caused her body to shut down had clicked back into its right place. She was smiling and claiming she was going to be okay. I thought the priest had put a drug in the Holy Communion and that she had lost touch with reality. For three days, she kept telling me that she was going to be okay. The puking seemed to have lessened but, apart from that, there was no visible improvement. I humored her again by pretending to agree. Defeatism and pessimism were what I was basking in.

She'd lost two babies, and Petros's future looked doubtful. She was dying herself, and yet still she held onto her beliefs. Go figure!

I believe that, through God, my wife survived. The blessing and Holy Communion saved her.

You may have heard someone say that a particular person married above his/her station—maybe they married someone especially pretty, wealthy or with a title before their name. This is bullshit! Remember that my views are extreme. In my opinion, you marry above your station when you marry someone of a better character than yours. I certainly knew I'd married above my station.

Coming face to face with such unyielding and unquestioning faith from someone special like Vas made me reconsider my views on religion. What if, for all my certainty, He existed after all? There was an overwhelming need to try.

I didn't know if there was a chapel at the hospital and nor did I care. Walking down the corridor, I found a bench and sat down. There was no chance of anyone disturbing me — everyone was avoiding me like the plague by now. I closed my eyes and pictured myself in church. I got on my knees (while sitting) and prayed like never before. I wanted to believe. I cannot remember how long I sat there. I asked God to save my wife and my son. There was a sense of warmth and belonging. It was so peaceful and serene that I wanted to stay there. The weight of the burdens I was carrying became lighter. The guilt lessened. The unbearable weight of hate and anger got lighter. Forgiveness was sought. I made a private pact with God and got up.

Even from her hospital bed, Vas was my beacon. It was because of her that I took the leap of faith.

The person who had sat down was different to the one who got up. I had accepted God into my heart. I guess that, however low you fall, He is gracious to accept you again and again. For this, I am thankful, for after seeing how bad I was, I don't think He should have given me a second chance. Lucky for me, He is merciful and forgiving. I found tolerance and love for my fellow humans. Not a lot, but I am on the right track.

One thing I can definitely say is this: up to that moment unless I was in Vas's room, I always felt a coldness in my whole being and a volcano of anger ready to erupt. When I got up, that coldness was almost gone, and I felt peaceful. Mind you, I was not ready to go and hug anyone and ask him/her to tell me their troubles. Baby steps!

Alongside Petros's incubator, there was another baby. I always called him 'Baby George'. For the first time ever I started talking to his parents, and we are still keeping in touch. Now this is a miracle!

I never went back to my deranged fantasy world of inflicting pain, and neither had I any wish for revenge in real life. The days and weeks following this episode, I prayed regularly. The way I can explain the difference in my life before and after is like this: there was order and peace in myself and my life; whereas before there was chaos, anger, hate, and vengeance.

Before all this happened I was an avid reader. This time, I had wisely chosen to fill my free time by resuming my passion with journeys to new fantasy worlds and complex thrillers. My one regret is not finding a single book dealing with infertility and IVF. It would have helped enormously reading someone else's journey. Oh well, I hope I do exactly this with this book.

Miraculously, a week later, Vas started accepting soups, and then, gradually, went to solids. That was the beginning of her slow road to recovery. The doctors still didn't know what had started it or cured it.

A few weeks later, Vas was able to leave that cursed room on her own two feet.

One evening, two weeks later after she'd fully recovered, we were visiting Petros. He was unsettled. The alarms kept blaring every five minutes. It was quite difficult seeing him in so much distress while not being able to do anything about it. Vas put her hand in the incubator, holding his little hand and, in between tears, would tell him, "You hang in there my treasure. Mummy is here. Please, don't give up. Continue fighting, and please stay alive. Please!"

That was not enough. The hospital alarms started blaring as well. One of the storage rooms on the top floor was on fire. Everyone was asked to exit the hospital immediately. We couldn't take Petros with us as he couldn't survive on his own. We had to leave him behind. How dreadful that was. Once outside, we saw thick black smoke coming out from the top windows. Would it get out of hand and burn the whole building down? I had found religion again, but I don't think I was ready to be tested. The fire engines were there in minutes.

Luckily, they contained the fire quickly and without any loss of life. Petros wasn't the only one who could not leave the hospital; other babies had been forced to stay in the same room as him, and other patients in other wards had similar problems. To my shame, not a thought was given for them. I only thought of Petros. If that had been a test from God, I had failed miserably (as usual).

We finally brought Petros home for the very first time, three-and-a-half months after he'd been born. Two days later, my wife heard a voice in her head telling her to check on Petros. She saved his life[18].

I am no longer an indifferent Christian. I believe! Sometimes I struggle, but I am on the right path. I no longer hate you or anyone else. Now that is a miracle!

I am not going to tell you anything else about faith in this chapter. You can draw any conclusion you like. Whether you believe or not is your own personal choice—exactly as it should be.

God bless you all!

---

[18] See chapter 17

CHAPTER SIXTEEN

<u>MISCARRIAGE OR LOSING A FETUS</u>

"We wanted to create life. I did not sign up for this."

From my blog: www.vaspx.com

Imagine if a woman who was four months pregnant had a miscarriage or had lost her baby because of various medical reasons before actually giving birth.

What would your reaction be? *It is not really a formed baby yet: it is a fetus.*

Being that it is a fetus, the parents should not be so devastated.

The baby didn't join his/her family alive in this world, so the loss for the family is not that great.

There was no bonding between the fetus and his/her parents, so they should be upset, but not as much as if they'd lost a living baby.

They should try for another one; once they have it, they will forget about the lost fetus.

Put it down to bad luck; forget about it, and move on.

The list is endless …

All of the above would probably have gone through my mind when I was single or if I had managed to have my family without complications. I would have been none the wiser and would have basked in ignorance and stupidity.

Why would someone get so upset at the loss of fetus?

Before you dismiss it, try imagining that you are living through the experience. Your own flesh and blood is unable to join you alive in this world. The experience of losing her precious baby shatters your glorious wife. While ignorant people like me think it is not that important, someone is living in a cesspit of depression, mourning, and devastation, their life in tatters, their faith shaken. This is how devastating the experience of losing a fetus can be for a couple. They don't dismiss it as bad luck. They don't just try again. They cry, and they mourn.

After going through the harrowing period of infertility, my wife got pregnant. A few months later, we lost the baby. It was out of our hands.

In those months, that fetus was the center of our lives. We talked to him daily, making plans with smiles on our faces. For us, he was not just a fetus. He was our son.

He was our flesh and blood. He was our life. Even though he was inside my wife, he had already taken his post in our family, becoming our beacon of hope. He was the catalyst for the world making sense again. After so many years of trying to get pregnant, we were finally a few months away from welcoming our son into this world, ready to nurture, guide, teach, and love him.

I cannot remember the times I heard my wife talk to him. There were too many. It was our daily thing.

Then the killer blow came: we had to lose him. We were a couple who battled with infertility and who needed help. With that help, we managed to take a step closer to achieving our miracle. To come so close to bringing our son home only to have him taken away from us was a hard pill to swallow.

Did I consider him a fetus?

Of course not! He is my son. He did not manage to join us alive in this hard world, but to me, he was not just a fetus. He is my flesh and blood, and we miss him dearly.

Seeing him come into this world without a life and holding him in my arms, knowing that it was only for a brief period, was devastating. We knew that we could not take him home. There was only one place for him: the cemetery!

We lost a piece of ourselves that day. The world did not make sense. Nothing did! I questioned the existence of a righteous God as anger took center-stage in my heart.

My wife was inconsolable, while I was basking in anger, depression, and hate.

Did I still think that it was not a big deal? Did I think

that I should not have been so upset, as he was only a fetus? Of course not.

I can understand why some people might think that. They have not experienced it. They have not lived through it. For them, someone outside their own bubble lost their fetus. It has no direct effect on them, so they look at it through tinted lenses.

They are wrong, just as I was back in the day.

I have learned my lesson the hard way. I hope no one else has to. Imagine learning the hard way by losing your unborn child.

For us though, that was not enough. We had the privilege of going through this soul-destroying experience a second time.

Do you still think that it is no big deal? Do you still think that it is just a fetus?

If you are ever in the presence of one of those tortured people who has lost a child, treat them with the respect they deserve. They have just lost their flesh and blood!

We suffered. We fought to achieve our miracle. We are VASPX.

CHAPTER SEVENTEEN

<u>DEATH</u>

"Where we wanted to create life, we encountered death and a fight for the survival of our very family."

Death and taxes come to us all. This clichéd phrase seems to be the only constant in our lives.

When you want to create life but face only death, it is something that you least expect and are unprepared for.

No words of comfort or religion can ease your pain. That was the case in my situation.

First IVF

My wife had to take a tablet to terminate the pregnancy when she was four months pregnant. As you know, she battled infertility for five years, and against all the odds, she got pregnant through IVF. To achieve this and to be told that the life we were trying to create was no more, was a hard pill to swallow.

Try living for four months thinking that at long last you will have a baby — and to then be told that you are childless again. If you were to have met me back then, you would have thought I was just a very quiet man (I never show any emotion and neither do I ever talk about my life). However, contrary to appearances my whole being was consumed by rage, anger and hate. A few swear words were the least of my problems, so cut me some slack. My life was still stuck in trying to have a baby but this time I had a dead baby. What a great a life I had. Nothingness. Do you get it now? These are the feelings that someone who goes through this experience might feel.

Burying Xristos at the cemetery was devastating. I did not want to go, for by not going, I hoped to make it untrue. It was a typical miserable English day—cloudy, cold, and with soft rain falling—appropriate for a burial. Vas, our priest, and I were the only ones there. Seeing the little coffin lowered to the ground and knowing that it was Xristos's permanent residence was just too much. It was as if time was moving in slow motion. I could see his little coffin going down inch by inch. It was torture. I wanted to grab it and take him home where he belonged. I was still hoping that at the last minute he was going to cry, indicating it was all a terrible mistake. The silence was deafening. When he was born, he was just like any baby, but smaller—there was no logical reason for me to expect him to cry. He was dead. I have witnessed him dead.

All I got instead was the priest saying whatever religious crap he felt like saying, which I did not understand or wish to hear. I'd only let him come for Vas. The only voice that I could hear crystal-clear was Vas's screams and sobs. I had to keep holding her, for sometimes her legs would crumple beneath her. I did not shed a tear, feeling I had to to be strong for her. She needed me. Reverting to my stoic persona, I was shredded to pieces inside. I never really mourned Xristos. What kind of a father did that make me? Not a good one, I can tell you that much!

I looked around at the headstones of dead babies, imagining it as colourful, with flowers and toys lying around. My son became a resident of the worst place on earth. He never got the chance to take his first breath, first step, nor utter his first word. Damn you all and your carefree lives. *I was the king!*

The only good thing was that there were no other relatives there to console us on that day. I would have taken my anger out on them. "I understand," "Have faith," would have been the common crap to come out of their mouths. At least I was spared that kind of anger. Of course, it would not have been their fault for trying to be supportive. They did not know that *I was the king.*

I left a bit of myself in that cemetery. Seeing my wife crushed and knowing I was unable to help her drove me to near madness. We went home and sat in silence. I knew that our house was a place where joy, laughter, and happiness departed on a one-way ticket, never to return. We were no longer three. All I could hear was Vas's crying. I saw my wife hit rock bottom. I thought my hate had already reached its zenith--boy was I wrong!

This is what was going through my mind: *I only wanted to be a dad. I did not sign up for this! I was not a soldier, where I knew I could face death at any time. This was a peaceful dream. This was a bloody dream to create life. Do you see the irony? Death was not part of the equation. Somebody made a mistake! Do you hear me? Are you deaf? Somebody made a mistake, I tell you! Give me my son back, damn you! Give me my son back.*

When I was younger, if I had heard of someone losing a baby, I would have shrugged and probably said, "Oh well, they can try again!"

Yes, this is how stupid I was.

After we lost Xristos, I was at a friend's house. I had a bottle of Glenmorangie keeping me company and a cigar in my mouth. I should not have gone, as I was in a very bad place. I totally blanked everyone, giving short, abrupt answers to whoever dared speak to me. I overheard one guy I had not seen for a long while talking about me. Let's call him Thomas.

Thomas: "What is the matter with Steve tonight? He is acting like a jerk. He is making no effort to talk, and he just ignored me."

John: "Shhh … his wife was pregnant, and they have lost their baby."

Thomas: "That is bad. They are young, though, they can try again. It is not as if it was a real baby."

John: "Shut up. He may hear you."

It was too late. I heard the idiot. It took all my strength to pretend I did not hear what he had just said. I wanted to break the bottle of whiskey over his head. I did not realize that Thomas was reacting exactly how I'd have reacted a few years back. I can see it now — he was only as stupid as I was. The only difference was that now I was on the receiving end.

The pain of losing your unborn baby is as real as it gets. You don't just dust yourself off and try again.

At home, I began to ignore our wounds. I could not bear seeing Vas so depressed. Being unable to do anything to help her made me feel a failure. My way of coping was to move forward. I showed no regard or compassion towards her. My rationale was that if she got pregnant again, she would be able to move past Xristos's death. *I was the king!*

With this in mind, I pushed her into the second IVF so soon. It didn't bloody work.

Was I surprised? No! Do I have regrets? Of course I have fucking regrets. I have regrets about the things I did and the things I didn't do.

It was after our **third attempt at IVF** (we had it five short months after Xristos died) when Vas finally became pregnant with twins that the real scares began.

At five-and-a-half months pregnant, Vas had an emergency caesarean. They pronounced Andrea dead. Another member of my family was dead because of our dream to create life. They placed her body on the counter to make room for Petros's arrival. My daughter discarded there, dead and forgotten, looked as if she had never mattered.

A few weeks later, Andrea was supposed to be transported to our local hospital. There was some mix-up with the forms, and our ambulance refused to come. Gillingham hospital asked me if I could drive Andrea instead. This was while Petros and Vas were fighting for their lives. Of course, I agreed.

Father and daughter were taking their first and last trip together. I put the little box she was lying in into the car. I could not help myself. I broke down and cried when I opened it. How do you ever manage to erase that picture from your mind? Your dead baby! Would you ever want it to be erased? What if you forgot her face? You are damned if you do and damned if you don't. I was damned already anyway.

Had all this happened because I drove Vas those two-hundred-and-twenty-five miles down to Margate? Was I the cause of this disaster all along? Was everyone I cared about doomed to die because they were in my life? Was I that cursed? So much hate! Yes, I was deranged. Why couldn't I be? I'd earned it. *I was the king!*

People take road trips singing and laughing with the music blaring. I was driving two hundred miles with my dead daughter lying in a box next to me. Can you see why I hated God and the rest of humanity?

I never forgot her face. Hers is the second hole in my heart. It was a very silent journey—I will never forget it, for all kind of terrible thoughts were going through my mind. I had only Vas and Petros left. Their continued existence did not look too good either. That was what my pathetic existence entailed at the time: keeping score of the dead and living members of my family while, all the while, I was in good health. I was terrified that I would be asked to make a second trip with Petros. These were unimaginably scary new heights, for it had the chance of happening twenty times a day. I was sure it would come when I least expected it, crushing me like an ant and taunting me for the insignificant being that I was. Having not been bothered at the beginning whether I even had kids, I did not deserve to have any now. I was my own worst enemy—I had so much free time and was always imagining and expecting the worst possible scenarios. If you'd met me back then, you would have thought that I was deranged. Inside, I was shaking like a leaf.

This is for you, the reader. For one minute, close your eyes and picture yourself in my place. After a long and horrible process, your wife gets pregnant, and you have lost your first child. She then gets pregnant with twins, and the first one dies. The second could die at any time. Your wife is dying in another hospital. All that you have in this miserable world resides in these two hospitals. Every day you think that this is the day you are going to lose it all. There is nothing you can do to make them get better. Every day they get worse. You just know that you are going to lose them. How are you holding on? Do you still have faith? Are you still feeling love towards your fellow human beings? Do you still believe that there is a just and benevolent God? I hope you do because I don't want you to make that descent to my kingdom. Never take the first wrong step. Nothing but ugliness awaits you.

If I had lost Vas and Petros, I would sell everything and disappear. Seeing anyone I knew would have reminded me of what I had and what I had lost. Why am I bringing this up? Because I had actually considered what course of action I was going to take. Imagine how basking in that kind of pessimism affected my being! With every day, the chances of my losing everyone were increasing. Petros was on a countdown. When Petros's countdown was over, Vas's countdown would begin.

Every night before I closed my eyes, I hoped (definitely not prayed) that they would both be alive when I awoke in the morning.

Going to sleep with that nightmare hanging over your head every night for weeks on end takes its toll on you. You never want to go to sleep, hoping that, if you stay awake, the miserable morning might never come. For that morning brings with it what you are most afraid of. What is the point of waking up to find out you are the only one standing, with the rest of your family dead?

I hated the mornings. The first thing I did, as soon as I opened my eyes, was to check that Vas was still alive. I did not reach over to hug, kiss, and wish her good morning. Next, I would call the other hospital to ensure Petros had survived the night as well.

I would sometimes violently shake her during the day while she was lying in the hospital bed. She would be moving around in discomfort, and I would listen to her grunts of pain. I would drift off to my hell; sometimes, after twenty minutes or maybe two hours, I could hear nothing nor see her move. All I could see was a lifeless body. I would rush to her, with my heart in my mouth, to shake her, calling her name, thinking she was dead.

"Vas ... Vas ..." I would scream.

To my relief, she would open her eyes in panic, wondering what was happening.

"Wh ...what is the matter?" she would ask.

"Sorry, I tripped and lost my balance," I would reply.

Vas could achieve sleep only through exhaustion or drugs. Her breathing was so shallow that I could not see her chest move. Always thinking the worst, I would scare her, waking from the little sleep she managed. Try living in that atmosphere of death every day; try watching your wife dying, knowing that you have failed her. It can make you do unimaginable evil things. I have seen the depths of my evil side. It was bottomless.

Would you have turned out to be a better human being than Iif faced with the same situation? It is a rhetorical question—there is no need to try to imagine this. It is one thing I would never wish anyone to experience. It breaks you and destroys whatever good is inside you. It changed me for the worse. I wanted it to stop, hoping it was just a nightmare, but it was fucking real. To my shame, I ended wishing that it visited someone else. I've had my fill of death. I'd had enough of trembling. I thought I was the only person in the world who was suffering at that time. I was delusional, which is why *I was the king!*

When I first started in business, I went through quite a few tough times. Money was often tight, and I'd struggle to pay my bills. At one stage, things got so bad that I thought I would lose it all. I honestly thought that it was the end of the world for me. Facing foreclosure on your home or business can be quite devastating.

It is nothing compared to facing the death of a member of your family. Home, cars, and money can be obtained again and again. Death is finite. This is when the real end of the world comes for anyone. No second chances; just complete annihilation. When you think that you could be the only one standing, is when the real madness begins.

I had the privilege of living through those feelings, knowing I was facing a future of loneliness. When someone gets divorced or loses his wife, given time, most find a new wife/partner and try for the second time to rebuild their lives. Not for me. With Vas gone, so would my heart. I've given it to her unreservedly, with no intention of sullying it by giving it to anyone else. Had I lost them both, no one would have ever been allowed to come close to me. I am committed, dedicated, and relentless. If I was told that the world was due to explode, I think I would have been the only one with a smile on his face. I welcomed death, for that would have put an end to my pain.

While Petros was still fighting for survival and Vas recovered, we were informed that Andrea was ready for burial. Going back home to bury her was déjà vu for us. Vas was in tears the whole time. Those four hundred miles (there and back) were very long. True to my form, I showed no emotion. How could I have cried when my wife needed me to be strong for her? Inside, I was an emotional wreck. I never had the chance to mourn Andrea's death, and here I was witnessing her burial. How could I have spared a second to mourn her death when Petros and Vas's lives were hanging by a threat? My life was unravelling, and I concentrated on the two that were still barely alive. She deserved at least that much from me. *I was the king!*

I stood there while they buried my daughter in a row of countless other babies. Seemingly stoic, I comforted my wife, while every ounce of my being was shedding tears inside. I wanted to cry! I wanted to scream! I wanted to talk to Andrea! I said and did nothing. I wanted it to be me going under instead so that Andrea would have the rest of her life to blossom into the amazing person I knew she would turn out to be. At least she had her brother Xristos to look after her.

We have been here before. Did that make it any easier? Hell no — if anything, it was even more devastating than before.

There are three things that I remember vividly:

- My utter devastation as they were lowering Andrea's coffin into the ground.
- My wife's constant crying.
- The higher number of dead babies in that section of the cemetery.

I was watching the film *Meet Joe Black* with Brad Pitt. Death calling around. Every time I watch it, it sends shivers down my spine. I must have seen it thirty times. In the film, Brad Pitt depicts death as something curious and bored. In our real life, death was dark, cold, and full of vengeance.

Well ...

What can I tell you? Was there anything I could have done that would have empowered me to face this catastrophe better?

Death is devastating. Everyone deals with it differently. Is there a right and wrong way? I don't think so. Personally, I found it soul-sucking — life came to have no meaning.

The one thing I could have done without was the efforts of my friends and family — too much talking, too much constant gesticulation. I suppose this is the Greek way.

In hindsight, I should have grieved and let the tears roll. There is nothing wrong with a man crying. I know that now. I should have screamed, smashed things, and dealt with the loss of my babies. I could've still been a strong shoulder for my wife while my tears were rolling. You see — emotionally I suffered from constipation. The thing is, I was taking one wrong step after another. It is no surprise I messed this one up as well.

As I've said, people have different methods of coping. Some people write a card on their dead baby's birthday. They might go to the cemetery and talk to him/her (Vas did a lot of that when we lost Xristos). I believe there is no magic formula. The only thing that I think makes it more bearable, providing you have other kids, is time. It is still painful, but after, say, a period of five to ten years, it is more manageable. Everyday life and concentrating on your other kids might make it easier to live with.

I guess the pain remains the same if you are unlucky, and

you don't have other kids. Every time you hold your niece or nephew or see any other baby for that matter, the floodgates of pain and loss open, overwhelming you. Depression, futility, anger, and resentment come in their purest form. You live with raw pain every day of your life until you die. You welcome death, hoping that it will be your way to be with your baby, as you had not been given a chance to hold him/her in this cruel and unjust world. This is how devastating it is.

For us, Mother's Day is quite difficult. Whenever Petros wishes Vas, "Happy Mother's Day mom," I can see the tears of joy and sadness roll down her cheeks. Petros was none the wiser when he was younger, but now he knows the mixed emotions Vas faces. We always go to the cemetery after we go for a meal and put flowers on our angels' graves.

I was talking to a friend of mine (John), who has three sons. There is a big age difference between the first and second. They lost their second baby and found it quite devastating. After reading our first book, he told me that having one son already made the pain more bearable.

Another lady told that she'd been pregnant with her first at the same time as her best friend. Sadly, she lost her child, which made it unbearable to see her friend and her baby. She would not answer the phone or open the door when she called. She became a hermit for a few years. She just could not bear to see or hold her friend's baby. Seeing them brought on an unbearable weight of injustice and anger. She could not help it. That tight friendship was destroyed because of it.

CHAPTER EIGHTEEN

<u>MY SHAME</u>

"The road to hell is paved with good intentions. I had taken that road willingly and with no regrets."

This book could not be considered complete without a discussion of my biggest shame. There is no point in trying to better yourself by learning from your mistakes if you don't acknowledge them fully. Accept them for what they are and learn from them. I found it quite tricky writing this section, as my shame was stopping me from putting everything down. I thought that you did not need to know the exact details. In the beginning, I approached it superficially, thus avoiding further pain and shame on my part. I persevered, and now you can read the full account. I hope that none of you sink this low.

How many times do you lie in a day, week, or month? Are they big or little lies?

Have you ever lied to your wife? Have you come back home at five in the morning only to tell your wife the next day that it had been one o'clock? When you've had ten pints of beer, have you told her you only had a couple? When you played cards and lost one thousand dollars, have you ever told her you won a hundred instead?

Did you feel bad when you told those lies?

With Vas, I found a connection. She is the one for me. I get on her nerves sometimes, but it works for us. I have found the person who is right for me, and I have no desire or inclination to find another.

We were at a party where the men gathered separately from the women. When we got home, Vas asked me why we were laughing so much. I told her we were talking about women, sex, and cars. One of the guys said that, back in the day, he'd kept going for three hours. Another one felt that he could better that by saying he had sex ten times in one night. The last one said when he goes to pee, he has to stand on a stool because his penis would otherwise touch the toilet. Apparently, it was that long! We were all laughing. Vas rolled her eyes. I never kept secrets from her. It was the basis of our marriage.

That was how we started and how I expected us to end.

I never lied, but I sometimes omitted things. I always told her afterwards and explained why I had not told her at the time.

When we first got married, a visit from her parents would always stress Vas out. She was under pressure as to what to cook because her father considers himself somewhat of a food connoisseur. The first couple of times they visited, he was a bit critical. Apparently, the food needed a bit more of this, a bit less of that. Vas would get upset, but I would say nothing as I knew her cooking to be excellent. True to his form, the next time he visited, he was critical and upset Vas once more. Later on, when I was alone with him, I had a frank chat with him. I told him that even if Vas's food was not edible, I expected him to eat it and compliment her. He knew I liked him, but I pointed out to him that such a recurrence would result in a falling out between us.

He laughingly asked me, "Great. I cannot voice my own opinions?"

To that, I replied, "Of course you can. You can voice them to me when we are alone if they are negative, but never to Vas."

When he saw that I was not smiling, he was taken aback.

"When you talk to Vas, I want nothing but positive coming out of your mouth," I continued in a firm voice.

We stared at each other until he looked away. Only then was I sure that he'd got my message. I am sure he was not impressed with my attitude. The next time we ate together, he actually praised Vas's cooking while giving me a glare and then a smile. Even though I was rude to him, deep down I think he realized that I would have never let anyone hurt Vas, whoever it might be. Since I was ready to confront her own father, I am sure he felt I would always be there for her. We actually became closer after that. I did not tell Vas until a couple of months later when I'd had a couple of whiskeys. She laughed. You see, I am not much of a drinker, and alcohol loosens my tongue.

Sometimes I did keep some things from Vas. When there was a problem at the shop, I would not tell her until the problem was sorted. I just did not want her to worry. They were temporary omissions—that was all!

When we first began to struggle with infertility, my lying began—I did not tell Vas about my frustration regarding the changes in our sex life. When you avoid telling your wife things that bother you, you don't deserve to have her in your life. I know it is extreme, but it is my personal view. I never told her and instead tried to rise to the occasion every time, while thinking that it was an unreasonable obsession on her part. She deserved to know what was going through my twisted mind. That failure in communication was my fault. That intentional omission was down to me. Had we managed to get pregnant at that time, I would have brushed it under the carpet, not giving it a second thought. We did not get pregnant though—our situation only got worse. However, I had taken the first wrong step, and our journey was far from over. *I was the king!*

During our numerous IVF attempts, I never once told Vas about my hang-up regarding my miniscule contribution to the process. I rationalized this second omission by reminding myself that she had enough to deal with. I thought I was protecting her. As you can see, the second lie follows the first quite easily.

In the grand scheme of things, those were lies that could have still been overlooked. After all, it was an intense period. The problem was that I had already taken the first wrong step. I had taken that slippery road, and there was nothing stopping me from following it for the rest of our long journey.

Well, I was not the king for nothing. I did not do things by half.

These first two lies were gradual occurrences. Time blurred their effects and my guilt, but the road was more slippery now. The bottom line was that I was a liar.

From here on you will read about my shame and about my failure to be a good husband.

I withheld the truth from Vas about Petros's condition during the first ten minutes of his life. It was intentional and unforgivable. I rationalized it by telling myself I was protecting her. I was not walking down that slippery road anymore. I was sliding down fast without any brakes. *I was the king!*

Vas saw Petros only once and realized that his future did not look good. She was unable to get out of bed and, later, admitted to another hospital. I think seeing Petros that very first time made her realize that she was going to bury her third child. Her body shut down, putting her next in line after Xristos and Andrea. For the first two days (while she was still in the same hospital as Petros) when I went to see him, I would tell her that there was no improvement. Her face was a picture of utter devastation. She could not go and see him, which only made matters worse. On the third day, she told me that unless she left that hospital, her next exit would be in a coffin. Hearing her say that, made me more agreeable, and we left early in the afternoon. The following morning, they urgently admitted her to the Queen Elizabeth, The Queen Mother Hospital in Margate, about thirty miles away. The way I saw it, it was the same bloody coffin ready to exit a different fucking hospital.

At about three o'clock in the afternoon of her first day in Margate Hospital, I left to go and see Petros. It was like a carnival, with alarms blaring and nurses running to stabilise him. This was not once or twice, but constant. Hope died for me that day. I knew that as soon as Vas found out that Petros had died, she would give up on life. Mentally and physically, she was in a fragile state. The consultant told me to prepare for the worst, as Petros was not stabilizing. The bottom line was that Petros could have died at any time. It could happen while we were having that bloody chat, while I was driving back to see my wife, or at any second. The consultant went out of his way to stress this. I understood the need for it, but I would not accept it. Accepting it meant the obliteration of my family.

You might think you understand what I mean. Maybe! These are the feelings I was experiencing: fear, panic, despair, anger, and hate. Add to this hopelessness, futility, and nothingness, and we are on the same page.

As I got in my car I felt crushed, utterly defeated. I drove to the hospital where Vas was. When I walked into the building passing down corridor after corridor leading onto a never ending room after room of sick people, I hardly noticed nor did I even glance at them. I couldn't care less about their troubles. I could smell that unique hospital scent that normally made me feel on edge. It had no effect on me now. I truly had the emotional capabilities of a robot. Eventually I turned the corner and there was the door to her room. Turning the corner, I reached Vas's room. The door handle was seized with a trembling hand. What could I tell her? I paused, too afraid to enter. However, whether I remained remained outside a minute or an hour, one way or the other, I had to go in.

She was just laying there, so deathly pale and as her eyes met mine I saw they were filled with an anguish and desperation that nearly pulled my heart out. Her longing to hear some good news about Petros was as evident as a hundred-foot-tall billboard. Leaving Petros to come face to face with the same deathly atmosphere was just too much. Our marriage had always been built on honesty, but at that moment I did something I felt ashamed of because it wasn't how I really felt; I smiled and then told my wife a complete lie.

I don't know why I smiled, but I did. Perhaps it was some kind of automatic defence system. Apparently when we smile, we produce endorphins; the body's natural pain killers. I was all too aware of the seemingly hopeless situation we were in. But I had to be strong for Vas's sake. Where there's life, there's hope.

She saw me smiling, thinking that I had good news. What would you have done? Would you have told your wife the truth or lied?

I opened my mouth, and the words poured out.

"Petros is hanging in there, and he is getting stronger."

The relief on her face was evident.

"I just knew it. I just knew he is a fighter," she said, in between pain and tears.

I felt so guilty for saying something that just wasn't true but I mustn't show it. How could I have done this? I had given her hope of life when it seemed to me that yet another death was the only certainty for us. I went totally cold inside. We were going to lose Petros as well. It was just a matter of time. Would it be hours or minutes, today or tomorrow until he joined his brother and sister? I didn't know. All I knew was that the time would come. Deep down I was hoping against hope. If Vas could hang in there a bit longer she might be able to pull through. Can you understand how inhuman that was and what a disgrace of a husband I was?

We had started by trying to create life, and it looked as if I was destined to be the only one left standing. No babies. No wife. Nothing. Yes, I felt all cold inside, but I had no regrets. I was trying to protect my wife from the truth. That was how my twisted mind rationalised it. The slippery road changed to a bottomless cliff. There was nothing stopping me now.

I intentionally failed her. Yes, I did not deserve to have her in my life.

At eight o'clock in the evening, I went to see Petros again. It was an oppressive scene, and there had been no improvement. Alarms still rang. I went back to spend the night in Vas's room. Dispirited and hopeless, I entered her room, but this time, the smile was intentional. The same lies came out my mouth.

Before I went to sleep, I called Petros's hospital to make sure that he was still alive. When I went back into Vas's room, the usual grin was on my face. She beamed.

"They are happy with the way he is progressing. He is getting stronger. It is your turn now," I said to her.

Total manipulation and dishonesty. I would look at her face, trying to quash the unbearable pain behind my false grin. It was strange. Here she was knocking on death's door, without once complaining. Women are made of stern stuff.

The lights were out. I was hoping Vas would be able to get some much-needed sleep. It was the worst time of the day for me. Sleep was out of the question. I spent the next couple of hours going over my actions. For most men, if they play over the things they did during the day, they might give themselves an imaginary pat on the back for the deal they clinched, the promotion they got, or their glorious performance during those passionate two minutes with their wives!

Liar. Liar. Liar. This was all I heard as I tried to sleep. *Would my Petros still be alive in the morning? Why did I lie to her? Would she survive the night?'*

I tossed and turned on the floor. The next time I opened my eyes, it was morning. Trembling with anxiety, I checked if Vas was still with us. It was about six o'clock. I could hear her grunting in pain. Phew! I called Petros's hospital to make sure that I was still a father.

They told me he could have died six times that night and to be prepared for the worst as there was no progress.

The call was made outside her room. I could not risk her overhearing the truth. The walk back was slow and hard.

I was thinking, "*Petros's chances of survival are non-existent. She should be made aware of that. But what if she gives up?*"

I entered, fully intending to let her know the truth.

It was like seeing someone gasping for air. Her longing to hear good news was that great. It was more than life itself. Whatever good intentions I'd had went out of the window. This was one room where the truth had no business. Even though I had lied to her three times already, she was still getting worse.

"They are happy with his progress, Come on, it is your turn now!" I said with a big smile on my face.

I could see a spark of life whenever I told her Petros was getting stronger. I was trying to change that spark to a raging fire. She just had to hang in there and survive.

Within days, she was thinner than she had been before she got pregnant. She could not eat, drink, or sleep. The deterioration was quick and drastic. The desperation to hear good news was all that I could see on her face. If she knew the truth, could she have done anything to influence Petros's recovery? No! She would have given up on life. With a smile on my face and a chuckle in my voice, I lied to her. *I was the king!*

At ten o'clock in the morning, I was at Petros's hospital. If I was hoping that the progress I had fabricated for Vas could have, by some twist in the cosmic balance, taken form, I was bitterly disappointed. I was met with the same shitty atmosphere. Petros was not going to make it. No part of him seemed to have formed. I was looking into the abyss. True to form, the consultant had another quiet chat with me.

Defeated and beaten, I set off to see my wife. In the meantime, my business was steadily going under as I was never there. Everything I had in the world was being snatched away from me. If I had any hair, I think I would have pulled it all out, for my fear of being left all alone was overwhelming. I could not help Petros, but I thought that I could save Vas. Talk about madness—but that is where I was headed. The usual lies came out. I had to convince her that he was progressing.

"You will not believe it. I saw his eyes today!"

I told her about his beautiful dark eyes. I was elevating selfishness to another level. She just had to hang in there.

All this happened in the first twenty-four hours after I'd unconsciously decided to lie to her. This was about four days after that frightening cesarean.

In the film *Groundhog Day*, Bill Murray has to relive the same day until he gets it right. In real life, there are no second chances. We reap what we sow.

Imagine having to live through those lies for one day. The next morning comes, and you have to say the same lies over again, this time with a few tweaks. You lie today because you hope that at least one of your loved ones will get better.

Tomorrow comes, and they are both worse. You lie again and hope that the next day you will get your lucky break. The next day comes, and it sucks as usual. This is the vicious cycle I was stuck in. I knew, though, that I was going to keep it up until one of them died. Only then would I stop, for, at that moment, everything would come crashing down on me. *I was the king!*

In hindsight, I see now that my problem was with those lies I was telling my wife. What would have happened if I'd had to tell Vas that Petros had died? It was not like the time I told her that I had painted the fence when I had not. I could have still painted the bloody fence. If Petros died, that was it!

She was dying. I felt that reality had no business venturing into her room. Who gave me the right to control what truths Vas could hear or cope with? Who gave me the right to manipulate her? For better or worse, I was her husband. I guess that was all the right I needed. I felt I was a failure and a fraud to both her and to Petros. Never have I lied so much in all my life. *I was the king!*

Before all this happened, if I was at work, I would always be on the phone to Vas and could not wait to finish and go home. We would stay up until two o'clock in the morning most nights, talking about everything and nothing. Very rarely, I went out without her.

Unfortunately, my lies brought this happy life crashing

down. For the first time ever, I dreaded seeing her, or, more accurately, I wanted and did not want to see her at the same time. After every call or visit to Petros's hospital, I would dread having to lie to her. Coming to this realization was a shock. I knew that I was failing her with my smiles and lies. To be in her room and in her presence was a privilege I did not deserve. How the hell do you ever get on with life with this noose hanging tight around your neck? How do you live with the knowledge that you are a fraud?

I dug my own grave all by myself, but it was not me who was dying.

The road to hell is paved with good intentions. I had taken that road willingly and with no regrets.

My fear was constant. I knew I could have received the dreaded call that Petros was dead at any second of any given day or night. I could have even received it while I was lying to Vas about his recovery. Every time I opened my mouth with the intention of lying, I felt the weight of the whole world on my shoulders. What could I possibly tell her if such materialized?

"You know how I have been telling you Petros was getting better? It was a lie. He is now dead! I only lied to protect you. I am so terribly sorry!"

No matter how I tweaked it, the end result was that I was a liar. It would have actually made Petros's death more difficult for Vas to come to terms with. She was expecting complete recovery on his part. I knew I was making things worse, but I just could not stop. By that time, there was nothing good inside me. I existed from one day to the next, knowing I had failed my wife. Can you imagine living with that kind of shame? Let me tell you, it breaks you up inside. It changes you, and not for the better.

It was not just those lies. She did not know that if by some miracle, Petros survived, there was a high probability that he would be a vegetable. I chose not to tell her. Who gave me the right to decide what information to dispense and what degree of truth it should entail?

Petros was getting worse, and I was lying again by telling her that he was getting better. Therefore, whoever died first, my lies would always haunt me.

Petros's death was inevitable. Being that I had a lot of free time on my hands, I actually tried to think how I could tell Vas gently that Petros was dead. This is how stupid I was. How can you find a gentle way to tell a mother that her son is dead? By that stage, I was so terror-stricken that, unknown to me, I think I was flirting with madness. No matter how I tried, I just could not find the right words.

What would her reaction be?

"I thought you said he was getting better. You are a *liar!*

Liar! Liar! You are a disgrace of a father and a husband. I never want to see you again."

Should I continue? My weird mind was going through all the possible scenarios. In every one of them, I was nothing but a liar. *I was the king!*

Some mornings, Vas was insistent that I called from her room. I could not refuse—I did not want to raise any suspicion. I always stood near the window, away from her bed, claiming that it was the only place I could get a good signal. The few times I agreed to do it, it went something like this:

Steve: "Hi, this is Petros's dad. How is he this morning?"

Nurse: "He's okay at the minute. You know his situation, though."

Steve: "Excellent!" (Here, I'd smile and wink at Vas. Vas would smile back.) "How did he get on last night?"

Nurse: "Not very well. He had quite a few episodes. The consultant was very concerned. He'll have a chat with you about it when you come."

Steve: "This is just brilliant. He is our little soldier. I bet he cannot wait to see his mother." Vas's face was a picture of happiness.

Nurse: "Excuse me? You didn't hear …"

Steve: "I have to go now. I shall see you in about an hour. Thank you very much."

I could tell that the nurse was confused. She either thought I was deaf or delusional.

Vas's grin was there, though. As far as she was concerned, Petros's recovery was a given. I was hoping the lie had given her a boost because, for all my bloody lies, she was still getting worse. The fact that those lies were killing me was irrelevant.

All the while, my visits to see Petros continued. The blaring sounds of his monitors were part of my life back then. I would hear them in my sleep. Babies admitted after Petros were going home in the arms of their happy parents. Petros had still not stabilized. *Where was the justice in that? Why couldn't we taste that feeling? Why did I have to keep lying to my wife?*

The other problem I had, which I did not know, was that by isolating and dismissing everyone from my life, I had no one to confide in. It suited me just fine at the time, as I felt I had no need to lean on anyone. My attitude towards well-wishers sharing their religious beliefs and empty words ensured my utter solitude. I thought I was smart, but I needed them—I was just too stupid and stubborn to see it.

When I argued with myself about the wisdom of my lying, my argument always won, as there was no one else to contradict that wisdom. Had I had the good sense to accept support and voice my lies, a good friend could have put me right, thus enabling me to see the error of my ways. I kept taking one bloody wrong step after another.

It was now the third week since I'd begun lying to Vas.

My panic went into overdrive. Vas had to fight — she just had to. I started talking to her about Petros getting stronger more than before. It was no longer just five times a day — it was non-stop. The only things I did not tell her was that he was now talking, running, or even driving a bloody car. However, if there was something feasible a premature baby could be doing, I told her Petros was doing it. That was how desperate I was. The dread escalated. I was ashamed of breathing, talking, and existing. I was ashamed of being me! *I was the king!*

I did not know which way to turn. The day of reckoning was getting closer — my lies were catching up with me. Yes, I was going to walk out of both hospitals all alone. It made me take a closer look at myself and see the emptiness in my life. I keep repeating that I was a failure as a husband and a father.

You will not get to understand the true meaning of this statement until you are faced with the loss of every member of your family, the shame of being a liar, and the regret for all the wrong steps you took. You'll feel the guilt of being healthy, while everyone around you is now dead; you'll find yourself shaking uncontrollably and will feel a tightness in your heart. Maybe it is a heart attack. You actually want it to be so — after all, you would no longer be the only one standing.

Vas knows that I am committed, dedicated, and relentless. She has other words for me: suffocating, irritating, and controlling. Since I am the one writing this book, I shall stick with my version- I think it flows better.

We were now at the end of the third week. Despite the barrage of tests the doctors had performed on Vas, they still did not know what had caused her body to shut down. She had not eaten or drunk anything for three whole weeks. She was not going to last much longer. Had she died, I would not have been able to tell the difference.

The next morning, I went to see Petros. He was having one of his touch-and-go days. The damn alarms were always blaring. The nurses would settle him but, as soon as they took two steps away, the alarms would start blaring again. I stayed for about two hours that day, for I refused to leave without knowing he had somehow stabilized. If he was to have died that day, I wanted to be there with him.

Questions gripped my heart in a vice. I wanted to scream at the nurses to save my son and my life, but not a word left my mouth. I was a mere spectator of my own pathetic life. Petros's condition was so bad that I could not tell if he was alive by looking at him—only the monitors showed any indication of his state. When they muted the blaring monitors, I realized I wouldn't know if he had just had his last heartbeat. I could have no longer been a father and I would have been none the wiser.

Try living in an environment like this and then you tell me what kind of a monster you become.

Five minutes passed, then ten… so on, I lost track of time. The nurses finally backed away. Petros seemed to have stabilized. The monitors were turned back on. The nurses had not taken even five steps away when they started blaring like crazy again. Petros jerked his little leg, and one of the needles popped out. Whatever its function, it was very important, and it had to be reinserted immediately. The nurses fought back panic — they could not find a vein. They had pierced him so much that the visible veins could not be used. Several doctors ran over. There were so many of them now that I could no longer see my son. I was not even a spectator anymore. I just lodged myself in the farthest corner out of everyone's way and trembled.

There were moments where I felt detached from the pandemonium as if I was watching a horror film. The realization would then kick in, and I'd be unable to breathe or stay standing for the trembling. I wanted the earth to open up and swallow me. They finally stopped; a smile on their faces. Petros had survived yet another episode. I looked at my watch. Almost two hours had passed. I was not smiling. Would he be so lucky and have enough strength to survive the next one? When would the next one be? How much punishment could his little body take before it gave up for good?

He won that battle, but would he live long enough to win the war?

The consultant wanted to have another quiet chat. What could he possibly tell me that I didn't already know? I was not in the right frame to listen to him, and Vas would have been going out of her mind because I was so late. He insisted.

"Petros is not progressing as I would have liked. He takes one step forward and two steps back."

Unbelievable! I had just seen what had happened. I just nodded, wanting this bloody chat over and done with.

"You have to realize that with this lack of progress, his chances of dying are increasing."

I just nodded again. I did not like the way this chat was going.

"As I told you last time, even if by some miracle he survives, he will still be facing a long and tough road ahead."

"I know."

"He might be a vegetable. If not, then he will most likely have development problems, breathing problems, walking and talking, learning difficulties."

Unbelievable! This is what was going through my head:

It was hard enough dealing with Petros's survival on a daily basis, and he was telling me about possible future scenarios. His death could have happened during that last episode or while we had that bloody chat. Let's deal with today's scare and wishfully think that he will live long enough to take him home. If he survives, then and only then, we can deal with all the possible developmental problems he might face. I am so bloody late, and Vas will be going out of her mind with worry.

"I know. Thank you for doing your best for Petros."

"We shall have another chat on your next visit."

In my head again: *Of course we will. Why would you not want to pile more crap on me and push me to breaking point? Bring it on. I have nothing else in my life. I was the king!*

Had Petros died, would I have been able to drive to my wife without crashing and killing myself? How could I have faced my wife? I got in my car with my hands trembling. Sitting there all alone, waiting for the trembling to subside, gave me a glimpse of my future. Loneliness, hate, emptiness, anger, and hate. Yes, hate is twice! What a future. I started the car and sped. Could I tell her the truth this time? Surely, I should do the right thing and prepare her for Petros's death. Enough was enough!

As soon as I entered Vas's room, I felt a huge hit of déjà vu. Different hospital, but death was still hovering around to claim his bounty. The first thing I saw was Vas's petrified look. That was the shell of the glorious woman I married. Deathly white, black rings around her eyes, and with no strength to even sit up. How many hours or days did she have? I could see the fear on her face. She expected bad news because I was so late. Truth had no business in that room as far as I was concerned. A cheery hello and a big smile on my face. My in-laws were there. I just grunted at them (it was the day my mother-in-law asked me about bringing the priest).

I was an expert at lying by then. Without missing a beat, I told her there had been a lot of traffic and that I'd stopped at a shop to buy a present for Petros, which I'd conveniently left in my car. Her face relaxed, and a smile formed. Another lie! My heart tightened. I started telling her the usual lies about Petros getting stronger. The thing was, If Vas died first, I wanted her to go thinking her wish was going to bear fruit. The fact that it was not true did not matter. At least she could have found some peace. *I was the king!*

Well …

What I should have done was had faith in Vas and told her the truth. She was stronger than I thought. As long as Petros was breathing, whether it was because of the ventilator or on his own, she would have fought to stay alive, just like any mother. What is the point of getting married if your wife cannot believe what comes out of your mouth? She was his mother and had every right to know the truth.

Never tell the first lie to your wife, no matter what

journey you are taking. You never know how bad it may turn out to be. Don't be like me!

You might think that what I did was understandable given our situation. I disagree! To my shock, a side effect of my lying was that for the first time ever, I actually did not want to see my wife. I did not want to see her five times a day. Can you imagine admitting this? Yes, I failed her big time. While Petros and Vas were knocking on death's door, I had to deal with those crap feelings. Just knowing I had them compounded the guilt even more. It crippled me emotionally, leaving me with an extremely short fuse. I took it out on everyone around me. To my shame, most of it was focused on my in-laws, as everyone else was too scared to come near me. My in-laws continued coming, were actually still nice to me when they had every right to shun me, for they would have rightly thought that I did not deserve their daughter.

Possible scenarios:

- They could have both died. You would have never heard of VASPX. I would have been living in a ghetto somewhere, spreading misery until I took my last breath, for I am dedicated.

- Petros could have died first. It would have been all over for us as a family. Vas would have followed him soon after. If she had not, she definitely would not have wanted to have anything to do with me. I would not have blamed her.

- Had only Petros survived, I would have ended up not being a good father to him. I am the type of person who would have tortured himself about those lies. Dealing with the emptiness of Vas no longer being there, compounded by the shame of lying to her until her last day, would have crippled me and rendered me unable to be the father Petros deserved to have. My shame would have prevented me from being there for him, for through no fault of his own, every time I looked at him (he looks like Vas), all I would have seen was the mirror of my shame. My being so consumed with guilt, even Petros would have picked up that there was something wrong with me. It would not have been a happy atmosphere.

If there had been no lies, I would have been able to deal with it somehow for Petros's sake. He would have had the father he deserved! I would have been sad, for I would miss Vas terribly, but I would have built a happy life with Petros for his sake.

What happened during that period was out of my control. I made things worse by taking actions, wrongly thinking I could alter the outcome. I guess I nurtured the illusion that I could bend the future to my will. I know it now, but back then, I had no one to point out my stupidity. I feel blessed because both Vas and Petros survived despite my lies and wrong steps. This was the only outcome that would have kept us together.

I gave this book to a few female friends to read. They all said that they understood why I did what I did. I was disappointed and shocked that I'd failed to explain precisely why my lying was wrong. There is no room for being understanding in a situation like this. *I was a liar.* The only way I could stress my mistake was to ask them to put themselves in my wife's position.

I asked them, "Imagine you are fighting death and all the while thinking that your baby is getting better. You know you are likely to die, but knowing your baby is going to survive empowers you to accept your fate with no regrets. Out of the blue, your husband tells you that your son is now dead. You were expecting complete recovery, and you are unprepared for his sudden death. He dares to tell you he is sorry he lied to you as if this will make it all better. You never got to say goodbye to your precious baby because he claimed he was protecting you from the truth. You are his equal partner in life and not a second-class citizen. Would you have been understanding then?" Most of the women agreed with me. One of them said, "I would have divorced the bastard and then killed him if he ever did a thing like this." I would not have been understanding either.

It is easy to feel empathy for someone who did something wrong, knowing his intentions were good. It also helps when you know his story had somehow had a positive outcome. But what if the outcome had been different? Live through that kind of sad story and then tell me if you are understanding.

CHAPTER NINETEEN

THE TELEPHONE AND WHY ANSWERING IT WAS ALWAYS BAD NEWS

"Ring, ring, ring... Full-scale panic! A sense of dread and doom hovers above."

A simple thing like the telephone ringing turned out to have a devastating effect on me.

How many times do you hear the phone ring in a day?

If Vas and Petros are with me, I can deal with the ringing. It's when they're not there that the terror kicks in. Full-scale panic, with my heart beating so fast that it is ready to take off, happens instantaneously.

At first, when those stupid people decided to call the house to find out whether Vas was pregnant, it was the ringtone I found irritating. My friends would call me at the shop, so I knew that when the house phone rang, it would only be someone who had five minutes to kill and a vague curiosity of whether Vas was pregnant. At that time, the ringtone only caused me anger. When I was at home, I would not answer it, letting Vas do it. After a while, I stopped her from answering the phone. The well-wisher on the phone had to deal with my abrupt, dismissive tone for only a short moment.

I started fearing that horrible ringtone after our third IVF attempt when my father-in-law called me three times. The first time was during the first night Vas stayed over at their house. She'd started bleeding heavily, and they rushed her to hospital. The second call was to tell me Vas had been urgently taken to another hospital, as she was bleeding and having contractions when she was about five months pregnant. As Vas was staying with them, telephone calls were the only means of communication. After his second call, I was dreading the phone ringing. It could have been a supplier or a customer, but until I found out who it was, I was a bag of nerves. The following week, Vas seemed to have stabilized. They said that they could discharge her by the end of the week. Instead of getting to see that, I received a third call from my father-in-law telling me that Vas had to have an emergency cesarean at five-and-a-half months pregnant. He could not help it, but hearing his voice on the other end of the line was like a stab in the heart. How I hated his voice back then. He is the kind of person who wishes peace and love in the world, but his calls were killing me.

One night, I was back home when Vas and Petros were fighting for their lives, and the phone rang. I sat up. It was two o'clock in the morning. I expected to hear my father-in-law's voice giving me more bad news. Instead, a friend of mine was out, having had a few too many beers. In his drunken stupor, he thought about calling me, telling me about the great time he was having. After I finished with him, he sobered up immediately. Idiot!

But it wasn't until we took Petros home that the phone indeed became an object of terror. I thought we were home free and so let my guard down. It only lasted two lousy days. Two whole days of basking in hope before terror showed up again.

While at the shop talking on the phone to a customer, the phone bleeped, but since I was on the extension, I could not see who was calling. I don't know why, but I felt uneasy. Uncharacteristically, I ended the conversation, immediately accepting the other call.

When I answered the phone, all I heard were screams from my wife.

"Steve … Steve …our baby … our baby …"

Those screams destroyed me. Hearing the pain, desperation, panic, and helplessness shook me to the core.

"Vas, what's wrong?" My legs were like jelly.

"Steve … our baby … Steve … our baby … " It was as if I hadn't spoken.

"Vas, hang up. Call the ambulance."

With dread and shaking hands, I put the phone down.

That telephone call broke me. Hearing my wife screaming like that was the lowest point in my life. I had somehow managed to deal with all the crappy things that had happened in our lives, but that call was the point I hit rock bottom. I felt I had lost the will to live.

Not knowing whether she had heard me or not, I dared not imagine what catastrophe was happening with Petros. I threw the keys to a member of the staff and rushed out with no explanation! By now, they knew that for me to do something like that, it must have been an emergency. I got in my car and called the ambulance. The shop was only seven minutes from the house, but one extremely long drive.

I drove like crazy, thinking that by the time I reached home, I would either no longer be a father or no longer a husband. Madness was inviting me. Voices made me want to turn the car to crash face-on into a wall. I couldn't breathe; I was trembling. I could not see for the tears I was forcing away. I had to appear calm and positive when I reached home. I could not let Vas see that I was worried.

Stupid! Stupid! Stupid! That's what I was. We were facing complete destruction again, and I was worried that Vas would think she could not lean on me. She never asked me to be like that. It was just my macho crap and me.

Arriving at the same time as the ambulance, I found what I had expected: total destruction. Madness was not just flirting with me anymore. It was giving me an honorary open invitation.

Vas was beside herself, looking like a crazy woman. I have never seen a crazy woman before, but Vas fit the bill of what I thought one would look like. Screaming, incoherent, and a mad glint in her eyes.

Petros was on the floor, motionless. His face was gray, his eyes bulging out. Seeing our baby like that, just two days after bringing him home, destroyed my whole being. The ambulance crew gave him oxygen and whisked him away. We followed close behind. Vas was hysterical. Was he already dead, or would he be dead by the time we reached the hospital? I had found religion, but that was too much—we were hovering over the abyss.

Following the ambulance was like being dragged under a car-crusher, knowing full-well that once the button was pressed, it was all over. My wife was sitting next to me, crying and rocking back and forth. They were rushing my son to the hospital, and we didn't know if he was dead or not. The ambulance tore through the red lights, and I drove after them like a lunatic.

You hear people say the clichéd phrases when they

experience something dramatic: "I would not wish it on my worst enemy."

I would have done so, for I knew it would have crushed him. At that time, I wished the shitty things we were experiencing upon everyone else but us. I was the king!

"It was so bad, I despaired."

In my opinion, true despair is when faced with the total destruction of your family. Add to that the guilt that you were probably the reason for their demise.

By the time we were allowed to enter the room Petros was being held in, we found a transformed child. His little body could not handle his immunization injections he'd had the day before. Had Vas not heard that voice in her head and checked on him, they would have classed it as another unexplained cot death.

This is what happened: While Petros was in the hospital, he was always lying on top of an apnea mat. It's function is to alert the nurses/doctors that there is a problem with the patient's breathing. If the patient does not breathe within a specified time it blares away alerting them. Obviously Petros was breathing at his own pace which the apnea mat found unacceptable and it was always blaring. When it was time for Petros to be discharged, Vas would not agree to leave the hospital without one. To cut a long story short, in the end the hospital gave in and gave us one. Petros's first night at home was like being in a carnival. The mat was blaring every hour with us jumping like crazy out of bed to check that he was okay. The following day Petros was lying in his bed. The apnea mat started blaring. Vas picked him up and checked him. He was okay. *She tried to feed him*, but he was restless. She let him rest on her chest for a while, to give him a break. *As I said before, Vas heard a voice in her head (which I believe was not of this world), "Check your son now!" Straightaway she checked him, and all she saw were his eyes bulging out, his face going gray, and he was lifeless. That was when she called me.*

A month later, the hospital wanted the apnea mat back. Yeah right! In order to get the mat back they put us in touch with a charity that makes portable monitors. This particular one was a lot smaller and was constantly attached to Petros wherever we went. Numerous times while in Church people would turn to us to see who was making that dreadful noise. I would totally ignore their looks and would in utter panic check Petros. Yep! He was smiling and in complete ignorance to the scares he was putting me through. Petros's breathing was still in contrast to the accepted parameters of the new apnea monitor. Vas didn't want us to have the monitor when we were out. She felt that Petros was okay. Of course I disagreed. We've kept it for more than a year before we gave it back. During that time the nights were very difficult. Every single night I would jump out of bed in terror as his monitor would start that wretched cacophony of screeching sounds but thankfully ending up finding him sleeping and comfortable. Some nights I would hear the bleeping in my sleep and of course as you can guess, I would rush to his room not realising there was no noise coming from the apnea monitor.

After Vas's last phone call, working at the shop was just unbearable. I receive about forty calls a day from suppliers and customers. I would tense when I heard the ringing and panic until I heard who was on the other end of the line. I instructed the staff that whoever was nearer to the phone should stop whatever they were doing to answer the phone immediately. Failure to do so would result in instant dismissal. They might have been in the middle of serving a customer, but if the phone rang, they had to stop to answer it. Period! It was not a good way to attract or keep customers (or staff!), but I was scared. (For the first time in my business life, I had high staff turnover. They found it intolerable working with me and knowing I could lash out at them for no reason.) I would stare at whoever answered the phone. If they looked at me straight away, it was bad news. Not answering the phone didn't make it any easier.

Every damn time I answered the phone, I expected to hear my wife screaming. It got so bad that I used to take the phone to the toilet. I still do. You might think it's silly and that I should've gotten over it by now, but it's easier said than done. Pray to God you never get to experience what I have. Even though I thought I was unaffected by the experience, I now realize that I am damaged goods.

Can you imagine what kind of torture it was, and still is? After all those years, I still tense up when it bloody rings. It is not as scary as it was before, but the fear and the rush to answer are still there.

My mobile rarely rings, which is just fine with me. As soon as the number of calls I receive increases, I change my number, only giving the new one to about fifteen people. Obviously, every couple of years, the list slowly grows, and the number of calls increases again. I change my number again and start over. I have now found a solution: I have two mobiles, and only Vas and Petros know the number for one of them.

In 2016 while I was at the shop before opening time, I went to the toilet. Of course, the phone was with me. It rang. Straight away, I checked the number. The number was withheld. I answered straight away. It was the producer of the Sally Pepper show from BBC Radio Derby. She wanted to invite us on the show to talk about *AIEWWTBCM*. While we were talking, she told me that she was having trouble hearing me. I could not tell her where I was!

Eighteen years later, and that wretched sound still paralyzes me.

I hate that sound with a passion. I just hate it!

CHAPTER TWENTY

MEN SUFFER TOO

Men suffer too was going to be the title of this book. However it would not have been appropriate for the story. It does deserve a chapter though.

I told you how I felt during the infertility times. My selfishness made that journey worse but I am sure a lot of men living through this, will feel a mild version of my feelings. They might look unaffected but in reality they suffer too. I never wanted or sought sympathy from anyone but I was feeling sorry for myself. That struggle was faced with tight lips, not once expressing my frustration. It was wrong which is why I guess couples living with infertility are three times more likely to divorce. I'd lived five years with this monster. Other couples live through it for longer. Appearances can be deceptive. When a man doesn't show his frustration, it doesn't mean that he is okay.

We then had three IVF attempts in a space of nine months resulting in two pregnancies. Within fourteen-and-a-half months Vas gave birth twice resulting in two dead babies while Petros and Vas's lives were hanging by a thread. I still didn't show any frustration or fear but inside I was suffering.

The fears and horrors I faced during Vas's IVF attempts and birth were real and coming at me like an avalanche. They just would not stop. Vas thought I was taking everything in my stride. She was wrong. I was wrong as well. She wasn't a mind-reader. She didn't know I was a liar. However, liar or not, I was suffering just like any other man would in my situation.

Living in that atmosphere changed me. It chipped away at my strength, optimism and hope until there was nothing left. How else could it have ended? Once a scare was dealt with, there were another two waiting to raise their ugly heads. There was no respite. I sometimes found myself trembling for no reason.

As a man, how did I suffer?

- I needed therapy (frustration, anger, hate, and jealousy).
- I needed counselling (grief and loss of faith).
- I needed support.
- I suffered from emotional constipation.

As men, a lot of us have been brought up with the mentality that 'men don't cry' (it is true in my case). I remember back when I was at school and a guy was crying after falling down a flight of stairs. He was made fun of by the others, calling him 'a girl', just because he was crying. As a guy, if you are scared you will be labelled 'a baby' if you show it. This is how I grew up anyway. This is why I think women deal with life's challenges better than men. They express what they feel. I believe that men suffer from constipation as far as sharing or showing their feelings.

Living through infertility affected me just like any other man. Add to that the horrors and fears of IVF, pregnancy and birth and I can categorically tell you that men suffer too.

Men have to learn:

* To share their feelings.

* It is okay to be scared.

* The world does not revolve around them.

* Things will happen in their lives that they will have no control.

* They can only do their best for their family.

* Deal with their misfortune by letting the tears roll, shout and get angry. In the end take a long, deep breath and face whatever they are dealing with a new resolve and determination.

Life has a way of sometimes rendering what we think is normal and easy as difficult or even unobtainable. When this happens (and it is a prolonged process), whether you accept it or not, it affects you.

What I found hard to deal with was my inability to help Vas. Talking to her about it, I tried to explain to her that it can be quite difficult for the husband as well. Trying to keep the business running, paying the bills and, at the same time, watching your family fighting a losing battle for survival can drive you crazy.

Yes, men suffer too!

CHAPTER TWENTY-ONE

<u>SALVATION</u>

"Had they not survived, then what you are reading here would have been the imaginary and wishful story in the mind of a deranged monster. Me!"

Much to my anger, the priest showed up with my mother-in-law. Vas was woken up and given the Holy Communion and blessing. What do you know! However stubborn and hateful I was, the Lord did save my family. He had not taken a day off, as I'd thought! He tested me, and even though my failure was epic, He is forgiving and merciful. A week later, Vas was on the slow road to recovery. Surprisingly, that was the beginning of my expulsion from my kingdom. I found God. I would like to think that was the beginning of my journey to rejoin the human race.

When I saw that Vas was getting much better, we checked into a hotel near the hospital caring for Petros. It made it easier for us to see him more often and gave us a chance to be by ourselves. It had been such a long time since we'd spent time alone. One particular day after we visited Petros, we went to

Bluewater, a shopping mall in Kent. As we were having lunch, Vas decided that I should open up.

I remember grinning. *Women and their sharing of feelings!*

She hadn't said anything up to that time, as she'd been busy worrying about Petros and staying alive herself. She knew, however, that during that time, I had never offloaded to anyone (well, apart from spreading misery and fear to all those around me, especially to her parents). She was concerned about how I'd handled my trip with Andrea.

She put her fork down, took my hand, looked me in the eyes and said, "I want you to share your feelings with me. You have bottled up enough things inside. Tell me about your trip with A … And … with Andrea."

She then burst into uncontrollable tears that she could not stop. People sitting next to our table were starting to give me dirty looks and were whispering to each other. They saw my hand was still across the table while Vas withdrew hers in order to wipe the tears. I just smiled. I reached out, squeezed her hand, and told her to let it all out. I knew it would be therapeutic.

The other diners thinking that I was the jerk who had just made his wife cry were of no concern to me. I had lived the past eighteen months with people rightly thinking I was a jerk. It was a nice change knowing that, for once, they were wrong.

I was in no hurry to share my feelings. Vas would have needed earplugs if I'd started and would have had to ask God for forgiveness on my behalf. That knowledge brought a bit of peace to my heart as well. For a long time after that incident, I wrongly thought that I was right to omit certain facts from Vas and to lie to her about Petros. If she couldn't handle even mentioning Andrea's name, how would she have taken the hard truth in the hospital? *I was the king!*

I never told her anything that day about my first and last trip with Andrea. She was just not ready to deal with my twisted mind, and I intended to tell no more lies.

I don't think I am emotionally stunted. I have emotions but only show them when I think Vas can deal with them.

A few years back, the big cooker caught fire at the shop, which could have burnt the whole building down and me with in it. Within seconds, everything was engulfed by fire and black smoke. The phone rang, and the caller display showed it was Vas. I immediately answered it in a cheerful tone (while the shop was on fire), asking her if I could call her back. I knew she thought the shop was busy. The fire engine came in minutes. After putting out the fire and cleaning the shop thoroughly, I went home. When I arrived home covered in black ash, Vas was distraught, but I downplayed the seriousness of the incident so as not to worry her, and so she wouldn't insist on my buying a new cooker!

Vas often tells me that I should have married someone a lot tougher than her. But what would be the point? She would not be Vas. Vas is sensitive, giving, witty, and a bit crazy at times, and that is why I married her—for the whole package. If Vas tried to change herself, she would stop being the woman with whom I fell in love. For better or worse! Besides, she is far more ballsy than she realizes. I see an abundance of strength in her, for I witness it every day. It is not how big you are that determines how strong you are. Because she does not want to talk about what happened, Vas does not realize that many women in her position would have despaired as well, or even, God forbid, have given up. She feels that she was weak during that period. How wrong she is! I thought I was strong, but my inability to deal with the situation turned me into an antisocial monster. I am sure many men in my situation would have been better human beings.

Dealt some shitty cards, Vas never complained. She never gave up. She stayed the course, keeping her faith. At the first sign of trouble, I disowned God, wishing we had never embarked on this adventure. Who was the stronger of the two of us? She battled on to the end, never faltering. By showing no emotion whatsoever, I thought I was a shoulder for her to lean on. Yes, Vas went through the motions of crying, feeling sorry for herself, and despairing, but she was *dealing* with her emotions. I, on the other hand, looked tough on the outside, but inside I was a wreck. Contrary to what Vas thinks, she dealt with our shitty situation much better than I did. She has been married to me for twenty-four years and has put up with my weird ways; it speaks volumes of her strength of character.

She suffered even after her discharge from the hospital. After Petros's birth, because she'd been in constant excruciating pain, she'd been unable to sleep. The only solution offered was to put her on a four-hourly dose of Pethodine. The drug reduced the pain, enabling her to fall asleep—so far so good. However, her dependence on the drug meant her body had forgotten how to fall asleep naturally. For countless long nights, she climbed the walls. I was again a spectator, a tired one at that, but in the grand scheme of things, it was not a big problem. It took her months to adjust to it but, for a change, it was not life-threatening.

I was more at peace with myself. A monster like me found religion in the end. Not a lot, but I am on the right track. I am no longer the indifferent Christian I was in my younger days. I believe that faith is a private matter and should stay that way. I found my way and am always happy to share my experience in a conversation, but I never ram my beliefs down anyone's throat. Faith should always be a personal choice.

Whatever your religion, make sure you practice it privately and peacefully.

A monster like me found tolerance, compassion, love, and understanding for others. I realised that the world did not revolve around me.

Of course, the only reason for my salvation was because Vas and Petros came home with me. If they had not, this book would be nothing more than the imaginary and wistful story of a deranged monster.

Several critical events began the chain reaction that landed us where we are today. This is the first time that I have realized this. At the time, I had more important things to consider. Later on, we were too scarred and damaged to relive our past. It is only now that I can see the events that took place.

Going to Professor Nicolaides was such an important event for us. I was running on empty by then; you could have knocked me down with a feather. If we had not gone to him at that time, I would not have been able to cope with what was coming at us. I know me! I know the dark thoughts that went through my mind. The beast would have been unleashed, without a chance of ever being put back in the cage. That boost in morale when I was feeling scared recharged my depleted reserves. As a result, when we went to keep our date with destiny and terror, I did not reach my full potential for evil. For this, I thank him.

Since I am talking about critical events, it would be remiss not to mention the doctor who told me that it would be better to let Petros die. He could have quite easily stopped and have been legally and morally justified. At that time, his call, I suppose, was the only logical thing to do. When I begged him to reconsider, he did not let his pride rule his head. Yes, he said that it was of no use, being better if we let him die. He took pity on me though and continued trying to revive Petros, whilst knowing that because of Petros's first ten minutes, chances were that, if by some miracle he survived, he would have been a vegetable. Even today, I can see the logic in his argument. Petros defied all expectations, fighting to survive and become the good young man he is today. The decision of that stranger who, against his professional, legal, and justified instincts, fought for Petros, affected all of our lives. I don't recall his name or even remember his face, but he saved Petros. By saving him, he saved Vas. By default, he saved me. He touched our lives. He was our guardian angel. God bless him and his family!

The thing that I found the hardest to live with was this: One minute I was a father and in the blink of an eye, I could have been no more. One minute I was a husband, and again, I could have been no more. Day after day and week after week I had to live with this fear. I was living with this noose round my neck, from a dream to become a father. If you include my mistakes and my shame in this equation, I am surprised I did not turn out to be worse.

Digesting these events, I am both thankful and remorseful, wanting to list the army of angels fighting for my family while I dared to feel all alone:

- The doctors and nurses who tirelessly fought to keep Petros alive.

- My mother-in-law who, by bringing the priest against my wishes, brought Vas onto the road to recovery. Enough said about this!

- Vas, who heard what I consider to be the voice of God in her head. Right or wrong, this is my opinion. Had she not checked Petros as the voice ordered, he would have died, becoming just another statistic.

- The doctors and nurses who helped Petros develop into a young man.

I had an army of people wishing to support me in my hour of need, yet all I had for them was hate, anger, and dismissal.

Whatever was meant to happen in my life was steadily

unfolding right in front of my eyes, yet I was too blind and stubborn to accept that the world did not revolve around me.

I had scores of little victories in our war, but I only concentrated on the defeats.

I am lucky to have married Vas. At the time, I felt I was a curse to everyone around me.

I acknowledge my shortcomings and limitations. I can honestly say that this experience has changed me for the better. I was quite cocky before all of this. This experience has knocked that cockiness out of me.

You must have heard the story of the man whose house was in a flood disaster and was in danger of drowning. People came to get him, and he refused to leave. Instead, as the water started to rise, he climbed on the roof of his house. Other rescuers came, first with a boat and then a helicopter, but still he refused claiming that God would save him. When he died, he asked God why He abandoned him in his hour of need. God told him, "I have sent people, a boat and a helicopter for you. The only thing you had to do was help yourself."

I am thankful Vas took the mineral supplements. I have never taken any tablets or minerals like this in my life. After witnessing what she went through, and the strength they gave her, I started taking them as well. We both do, and they are the

'Nordic Naturals'[19]. Yes, we are helping ourselves. They are manufactured in America and they are available worldwide.

You cannot face your struggle hoping God will help you see it through. You have to help yourself. Your body is your temple. Keep it running like a well-oiled machine, with the hope that it can cope with difficulties and reduce sickness. If you are thinking of trying to get pregnant and you are not taking mineral supplements already, talk to your doctor and start as soon as possible. Pregnancy can bring so many unexpected terrors. The woman's body has to be as fit as humanly possible.

Many people who read *AIEWWTBCM* told us that they thought that we were brave to have survived this ordeal. How far from the truth this is! It was either soldier on or sink and die—not much of a choice. It was a mercy that we did not have time to stop to take stock of how dire our situation was. We were on autopilot. Yesterday it was that, today it was this, and tomorrow it would be another shitty thing—that was simply how our days unfolded. We instinctively fought to survive, taking it day by day, just like any one of you would have done.

Xristos, Andrea, Petros, and Vas were, and always will be, my salvation.

---

[19]https://www.nordicnaturals.com/professionals.php

CHAPTER TWENTY-TWO

<u>THE LATER YEARS</u>

"The fact that I survived it physically does not mean that everything is fine."

Petros fought and stayed alive, proving his old man wrong. Now we had to actually deal with all those hypothetical and highly likely scenarios the doctors warned us about; Petros could be a vegetable, have development problems, and/or have learning difficulties—take your pick! When their warnings materialized, it was quite daunting, as only then did I accept that my child would be disabled. Only then did I get to realize what a big mountain we still had to climb.

Petros would not burp easily. I would give him his bottle of milk every night about one or two o'clock in the morning. The number of times he threw up on me were countless.

He was diagnosed as having severe deafness. Vas, my beacon, was relentless. She would put her mouth near his ear and talk to him constantly. So much so that even a deaf baby would get a headache. She never gave up, even though she was getting no response from Petros.

The visits to the hospital continued. Vas's insistent

talking went on for months. A normal person would have given up. Not Vas! Eventually, he uttered his first word: "Dada." I think he picked me out first to punish her for the continuous headache. Just barely, he could hear. There was a spark, and Vas wanted to kindle it until it was a raging fire. Petros's headache increased as Vas started talking to him even more.

At the time when other babies his age were crawling or walking, Petros struggled to even sit—his body was wobbly, and he constantly tilted to one side. Yes, the doctors' warnings materialized. So much worry and pressure. He was fourteen months old when he started to crawl. Not walk, crawl!

At parties or weddings, babies a lot younger than he ran around, laughing and playing. At twenty months old, I was still holding him. A few people felt that we were overprotective by not letting him run around with the other kids. Run … were they taking the mickey? I was too tired to explain to them why I was holding him.

One day, Vas called me screaming. I froze, unable to hear what she was saying. My legs were like jelly. Something terrible must have happened again. I was shaking and feeling petrified. Strangely, I heard laughter towards the end. I asked her to calm down and to tell me slowly what was wrong. Laughingly, she told me that Petros had taken his first steps.

Not wanting to tell her the reason, I asked her never to

call me again screaming. It took my poor heart three hours to calm down. Living through that first call from her had shaken me to the core. My brain only heard the screams. It was not until a few years later that I told her about it. Petros was twenty-two months old when he finally started walking.

Trying to make Petros keep the hearing aids in his ears was a daily battle. He just did not like them and would pull them straight out. Vas put a sticky tape, attaching one side to his hair. It did not deter him, resulting in a hairless patch behind his ears.

He had to wear glasses, which he did not mind, but his size was such a worry for me. He was so small for his age.

One thing that kept us going was his smile. He was such a happy baby.

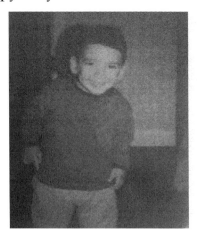

I so much wanted us to be a normal family. I so much wanted us to have a boring life, without all the highs and lows. Petros conquered his adversities in his own time; he would not be rushed. I was growing too. For the first time since Vas had been pregnant, the facial expression Vas saw on my face truly reflected what I was feeling.

We survived it and came back as a family. Andrea and Xristos never had a chance. We miss them terribly. They are forever in our hearts.

The fact that we survived it physically does not mean that everything was fine.

Vas still gets nightmares about that time. Even after years, she is still haunted by what she went through.

I felt that I was unaffected—sure, I'd gone through anger, hate, lies, loss of faith, and dismissal of others, but I thought it was no big deal. I was strong. Yes, we had somehow survived our hell, and except for my brief existence as the king of a deranged land, I thought that since I had not suffered physically like Vas, that I was alright. How far from the truth that is!

You have to ask Petros about this. Every morning, Petros and I would have breakfast together. If he wanted cereal, I would fill the bowl, expecting him to finish it. Halfway through, he would stop, telling me that he was full. I would then ask him to have another five spoonfuls. He knew from experience that any attempt to negotiate the number would result in an increase. He would have them, and then I would ask him to have another three since the last three had really not been full. He would complain and sigh, but I made sure he finished his bowl. He was still very small, and I thought if he did not eat enough, he would not grow bigger. Bless him, he suffered!

I have never let him have a sleepover. The thought of him being away from us was out of the question. I told him that if any of his friends wanted to stay over, it was not a problem, but having him stay away was a non-starter. Vas did not mind, but I never agreed. When we went to see my in-laws with the view of going somewhere with Vas for a couple of days, I would tell my mother-in-law that Petros should never leave her sight. If she was visiting any of her relatives, Petros should be with her. When she left, he had to leave, too. When I called to see how Petros was, I expected him to be available so I could talk to him. She had met deranged Steve, hated him with a passion, and had no wish to meet him again. Petros was obviously upset that he could not stay to play with his cousins, but the thought of Petros being anywhere that I could not get in touch with him was unacceptable. Yes, I was scarred and damaged! I was the king, even now!

I'd thought that I was going to lose them both, and I have never lost that fear. I don't think I ever will. I became overprotective of both of them. Vas thinks that describing me as "overprotective" is to undersell me—she thinks that "suffocating" is the right word! Well, maybe I am. Perhaps, if she ever reads this book, she will understand finally the full extent of the fears I have lived with. I was wrong not to share them before, but *I was the king.*

There are books about how to cook, lose weight, or assemble an engine. I wish I could have found a book about dealing with your child's illnesses. Even a minor cold petrified me, as his hearing would become even worse. Whenever I spoke to him, he had to move so close to me that his ear was actually a hair's breadth from my mouth. Every time this happened, I was forever worrying that his hearing would not return. When Petros had a fever, it paralyzed me. Since he was so small for his age, it took him ages to get over it.

When I was a teenager myself, I liked playing chess with my brother. One night, we played a couple of games that he won. We went to bed. An hour went by, and I could not go to sleep. I just could not relax knowing that I'd lost. I woke my brother up, asking him to play another game. My brother is two years older than I and a very peaceful person. He won again. Fuming, I went back to bed. It was a school night. At two o'clock in the morning, it was still playing on my mind. I woke him up. He did not want to play, but he could tell that I was not going to let it go. Instead of having an argument, he agreed to play, but only if I promised that it was to be the last game. I won. I then went straight to bed, and yes, I fell asleep straight away. In the morning over breakfast, I heard him telling my mom that he'd let me win because he knew that even though I'd promised that it would be the last game, I wouldn't let it go if I'd lost. He refused to play chess with me again.

When Petros was five years old, I decided to teach him how to play chess. I'd best get it out of the way now: I am not a good player, but I enjoy the game. Vas refused to learn as she finds it incredibly dull. I was showing Petros the moves, which he surprisingly picked up straight away. To encourage him, for the first few games I made bad moves so that he could take my pieces. He was proudly stacking them in line next to the chessboard and could not wait until he got the next one. Just to show him that he had to play carefully, I decided to capture one of his pawns. I could not have foreseen his reaction.

In a businesslike tone, he told me: "Put it back."

"You cannot just get my pieces," I told him. "You are bound to lose some of yours."

My comment was ignored, and he said again, "No! Put it back!" Where was the "please" I'd taken care to teach him?

I smiled, "No Petros. You can't just take my pieces. I am bound to take some of yours."

He stared at me and I stared back. What would his next move be? Would he learn the lesson about thinking before he made a move? Would he learn to accept that he was bound to lose some pieces before I let him win?

I didn't have to wait long. In a sudden move, he reached out, whacked all the pieces off the chessboard, jumped off the settee, and stormed off in a strop.

Vas told him off for behaving so badly, but Petros was confused. He looked at me, almost falling off my chair from uncontrollable laughter. He was only five years old! I was laughing even more when I told Vas later that I dreaded to think how he would have reacted if he'd lost the game.

An irritating hassle we had to deal with was when we met up with other Greek-Cypriots or when we went on holiday to Cyprus. I could see the disapproval on their faces when they tried to talk to Petros in Greek. "Oh, you have not taught him to speak Greek?"

As you know, we were an infertile couple who with the grace of God managed to have a child. We were in constant worry regarding any developmental problems, and we still had not reached the stage of learning difficulties. To say that we were terrified is an understatement.   He had enough to deal with. I felt it was irresponsible to pile more Due to the high possibility of learning problems arising, we did not want to put unnecessary pressure on him. We were not out of the woods yet. Our priority was for him to cope with the school challenges. He could have learned the language when he was older. It wasn't the end of the world.

After the hundredth or so time, I just lost it. There are so many times that you can explain yourself without getting angry with people who feel they know better than you. All they saw in front of them was a normal looking child. He was a three and a half months premature baby, with the worst possible start in life. They would tell me that a nephew of theirs was speaking Greek at the age of three even though he was born in England. I told you before how I reacted when Greek- Cypriots told stories about someone they knew who had the same problems as me. To my shame, being civil with my fellow human beings was lost for those fifteen seconds.

With a sharp voice and an angry glare, "I don't want him to learn Greek. Is it okay with you?" *I was the king!*

Unfortunate busybody, "Yes, it's okay. I was just asking. Sorry."

I was in no mood to explain to anyone with a disapproving look why Petros could not speak Greek. I was always next to him and interpreted whatever anyone said to him. Apparently, it was not enough for them.

When Petros was invited on trips at junior school, I always asked Vas to put her name down as one of the volunteers. The thought of Petros going somewhere without at least one of us with him was terrifying.

Petros's school years were a tough time for all of us. If I heard that anyone had picked on him or upset him, I threw myself down the warpath. During his lunch break, a canteen woman used to pick on him for being a slow eater. Immediately, I wrote a letter to the principal, threatening him and the school with litigation. We had a meeting where in a very sharp tone I told him that if that woman as much as looked at my son, never mind talked to him, I would sue everybody within reach. Petros was upset when I told him what had happened. He had a chat with Vas, asking her to deal with any future problems instead of me. Vas told me about the conversation, so I said to Petros that he could still confide in me without any fear that I would interfere. I would only do so if Vas could not sort the problem out herself. He was just seven years old, and my reactions had not been constructive. Living for so long with the fear of him not surviving had made me overprotective. Yes, I was damaged.

When he was ten years old, I took Vas and Petros to The Fat Duck, a restaurant just outside of London, for Vas's birthday. When we entered the restaurant, other diners turned to look at us. Petros turned around and told me with a grin on his face, "Dad, you are famous. Everybody is looking at us."

After having a good look around, I smiled, telling him, "No mate. They are looking at me because they are wondering what kind of idiot brings a ten-year-old to a place like this."

Petros was the only kid there, as it is very expensive. During one of the courses, they brought us each an iPod so we could hear music that complemented the dish. I guess for the money I had to pay, it was the least they could do.

After the dish was finished, the waiter picked up only two of the iPods, leaving Petros's behind. Petros wishfully thought it was his to take home. He asked me if he could take it, and I said no. Petros insisted, so to shut him up, I told him to ask the waiter, who I was sure was going to say no. He did, and the waiter actually said yes. In a split second, Petros put the iPod in his pocket, grinning. I asked him to put it back on the table, calling the waiter over again. I asked him again to make sure he'd understood the question. Of course, he said no. Petros's grin disappeared.

When we go on holiday, at night Vas will go to bed while Petros and I sit on the balcony, talking about everything and nothing until three or four o'clock in the morning. When he runs out of things to say, he will always ask me about the period when he was born. I think this topic is always his backup for when he does not want to go to bed. His mouth always stays open as I finish the story. I have told him this story so many times that he must know it by heart. He always laughs when I reach the stage where I was obnoxious to other people. Even though I always explain to him that I was wrong, he still finds it funny. Teenagers! The other thing he finds hilarious is the idea that I was terrified by the priest entering the room.

We were on holiday in Cyprus visiting my parents. Petros was twelve years old. My dad asked me to get him a beer. There were two brands. I shouted out in Greek. "Petro, which one do you want?"

The custom in Cyprus is for the first born son to be named after the husband's father. Also, my Greek name is Stelios.

Petros, "What did you say dad?"

My dad, "The KEO beer."

When I went back to the table, Petros repeated his question.

"I was talking to my dad, mate, and not you."

"You call your dad by his first name? This is so cool."

This is something that my eldest sister started when I was thirteen. My parents actually liked the fact we were all calling them by their first name. Petros was right. It was cool!

The following day, we visited my parents again. I was at the back talking to my dad. Petros was in the house and was trying to catch my eye. Before I asked him what he wanted, I heard him shout, "Stelio, I want to ask you something."

I looked behind me to see if my cousin Stelios showed up without me seeing him. There was no one there. I thought that I had most probably misheard the name.

"Petro, who are you talking to?"

"I was calling you, Dad!"

After I interpreted my conversation to my dad, he laughingly said, "The apple does not fall far from the tree."

I was not impressed, though. I went over to Petros, and out of anyone's earshot, I asked him why he called me by my first name.

"I think it's cool. Being that you do it with your dad, I want to call you by your name as well."

"It may be cool for you, mate, but the only name you will use when you call me is 'dad'."

"But Dad …"

"There are no 'buts' here, Petro. This is not up for debate."

Petros would not let it go for a while, but he got over it. He is relentless like his dad.

He does not get that all I wanted was to be a dad. Against all odds, I managed to become one. I earned that title, and this is the only way Petros can address me.

When Petros was thirteen and on a school holiday, he would ask me if he could stay up late.

"Okay, you can stay up until one o'clock."

"Come on dad. I am thirteen now. Let's make it two."

After getting my consent, Petros would go into his room. He always left his door open. One night while my in-laws were visiting, about one-thirty in the morning, I heard a shouting match. Andrew was shouting at Petros for being awake at that time.

Petros was trying to defend his corner, "I asked my dad, and he said it's okay."

To that Andrew told him, "You go to sleep right away, and I shall sort your dad in the morning."

Vas and I heard the heated exchange and sniggered.

Petros closed his laptop, got up and came into our room ready to complain about the injustice. I smiled and told him to go to sleep.

"But dad, I have another half an hour yet."

"It's okay. It is quite late, and by the sounds of it, your granddad is upset."

The following night (and until now), Petros has kept his bedroom door shut.

As you know Petros was put on the HFOV (ventilator). Every couple of years we are asked by the team of the UKOS trial to go to London, where Petros is faced with a barrage of tests. This is to keep a record of how babies who have used this ventilator, have progressed later on in life. He is exhausted by the time they finish with him.

Three years ago, while we were on holiday, we went on a Jet Ski (due to Petros's age, we had to be together). He was at the front driving, and I was at the back, holding on to him. He went quite far out so that we would not hit anyone. He was excited and decided that the laws of gravity should not apply to this particular Jet Ski. I understood his excitement and let him go at whatever speed he wanted. He was a teenager after all, and, though he can't believe it, I was one once too. He was tearing through the waves, willing the craft to take off. Every time it hit a wave, we'd jump into the air for a few seconds but then plunge down, with me hitting my head on his back. He couldn't stop laughing. I was holding on for dear life. Finally, the inevitable happened. We hit a massive wave and flew high into the air before gravity defied Petros, and we plunged down hard. My heart was in my mouth. I reached for the handles, trying to hold on to something solid, and at the same time, squeezing Petros between my arms and legs. My fingers got hold of the handles while my little finger touched the throttle wire. I held on to it with such force that it came off.

The Jet Ski flopped like a dead fish and ground to a halt.

Petros looked at me in alarm. "Dad, no one knows where we are."

"It's okay," I said. "The guy will come looking for us."

"What happens if he does not find us? I cannot see anything

apart from the water. I cannot even see the hotel."

"In ten minutes, our time will be up. He will probably give us another five minutes, and then he will come looking for us."

I had a smile on my face to stop him from worrying— well, that and it was nice to finally have some peace and quiet.

Twenty minutes later, Petros turned to me again.

"He is not coming. No one will find us," he said.

"Can you see the black dot over there?"

Petros nodded.

"That is him coming."

Five minutes passed.

"It is not him. It is just a black dot on the water."

"Oh, yes, it's him," I said. "The dot is getting bigger."

He finally reached us, and we had to be towed back to shore.

Petros still brags about the incident.

Last year, Petros asked me to go to the supermarket near where I work. He wanted me to buy hairspray. I have never bought one in my life. I told him to wait until the morning so he could go with his mom. He insisted as he wanted his hair to be just right when he went to school. To cut a long story short, I finally gave in. At the supermarket, I started going through the aisles and, unable to find the spray he'd asked for, I asked an assistant. Her first reaction was to look at my bald head and then smile. I was fuming at Petros. How cruel of him to send a bald man to buy him hairspray! He almost wet himself from laughing when I told him what had happened.

When I watch a film, I don't talk and don't like anyone talking to me. Vas hasn't got the same taste in films as me. So she will either watch it whilst being bored or leave and do something else. A few years back, I noticed that she started asking a lot of questions when I was watching a film. I would pause the film and deal with her question. I would then continue watching the film. She would start with the questions again. I would pause yet again. I would finally give up and turn the telly off without watching the film just because she wanted to talk. The only difference now is when I want to watch something I really like, I wait until she is asleep or out. It is inconvenient, but it is a real pain trying to watch a full film that she does not like.

I do something weird which gets on Vas's nerves. When we are watching something, and she has to leave for five minutes, I pause the telly and wait until she comes back. I don't want her to miss what we've been watching. When it is the three of us, she does not mind. She thinks what I do is 'cute'. Personally, I would have preferred a different word. When it's a room full of people, she gets angry with me. When we are at someone else's house, she is furious when I grab the control and pause the telly.

We were watching 'Man on fire' with Denzel Washington. Andrew (my father-in-law), got bored with the film and asked Vas for a cup of tea. Vas got up to do it. John asked Frank a question about his car.

Frank, "Shut up John. We're at the good bit now. Ask me later."

John, "You won't be watching the film for at least five minutes mate."

"Why?"

John, "Look at the telly."

I paused the telly and put the remote in my pocket. Frank had to wait until Vas got back.

Frank, "Is Steve for real?"

John, "This is nothing. He does the same thing in my own house. We all scream at Vas if she gets up while we are watching something."

They just don't get it, including Vas. She is my wife.

Period! If we have guests, she makes sure the telly is off. I also noticed that lately when we visit people who know me quite well, their telly is off. Oh well!

Vas and I have been watching 'The big bang theory' for some time now. It is late at night when it is on. Countless times, Petros comes into our room at two o'clock in the morning asking us to stop laughing

because we have woken him up. He rolls his eyes and actually tells us to go to sleep. If we don't continue laughing after it finishes, we laugh about something else. The older we get, the later we tend to go sleep, much to Petros's disapproval.

He is training to be a barber.

Petros and I were in the back yard lighting up the barbeque the other day. He had a serious look on his face.

"Dad," he said, "do you think God really exists?"

"Yes," I replied.

"How can you be sure? Where is the proof?"

"I am staring at the proof mate," I said, looking straight at him.

Petros was not impressed. "I know all that. What if there is really no God, and we waste our lives believing in someone who does not exist?"

He'd really picked the wrong person to talk to about religion. Vas was out shopping and could not come to my rescue.

"When I was your age, I was an indifferent Christian. I then progressed to not believing in God and decided, on the off-chance he existed, that I hated him. Looking at your mom holding onto her faith when everything was crumbling around us encouraged me to take that leap of faith."

Petros interrupted me: "But where is the evidence and undisputed proof?"

I was out of my depth. Believing in God was something that I'd achieved in the mayhem of trying to see my family survive. I have never talked about religion to anyone else before. How could I explain religion to a teenager who wanted to be entirely sure God existed? Why did he not ask me about cars or girls?

"Let us for one minute assume that He does not exist. Even if you spend your life following the Ten Commandments—don't kill, love your neighbour, don't lie, etcetera—by default, you will live your life being a good person. You have not actually lost anything. To believe, you have to be willing to take that leap of faith. Personally, I believe He exists for everyone on this planet. Whatever name He is given does not matter—after all, the teachings are similar in all religions. Love and peace. It gets distorted when you involve the human element. You get leaders of countries who become dictators, others who take personal selfish actions hoping that they will be remembered. They interpret religion to suit their goals. As human beings, we have free will, but unfortunately, we are also greedy. Power, self-importance, and money take center-stage."

Strangely, Petros smiled.

I went on. "Instead of people concentrating on what is important, they waste their lives trying to acquire power and wealth. They behave as if they are going to live forever. They end up having a lot of ex-wives and kids who want nothing to do with them as they were never there. Family, love, and peace are the essentials in life."

"Have you had a couple of whiskeys already?"

"Yes. Am I talking too much?"

"I only asked you if God existed. Instead, you had a rant about humanity."

I smiled. "It is always better to ask your mom about religion."

When Petros was younger, he would always call me at around 7:30 every night to wish me goodnight. He was obsessed with football and would spend ages telling me about footballers I didn't know. At weekends or during holidays, he would always be at the window, waving to me with a smile on his face as I pulled into the drive. I would look forward to it on my way home.

He is eighteen now, and there is no more waving from the window. I miss that dearly. I wish he was still my little boy. He is growing up and will fly the nest soon. I shall accept it, but that does not mean I must like it. Being a husband and father is what defines me. In the years to come, I hope he always seeks my guidance and friendship.

He wears hearing aids in both ears, and his hearing is just below normal level. He wears glasses and recently started wearing contact lenses.

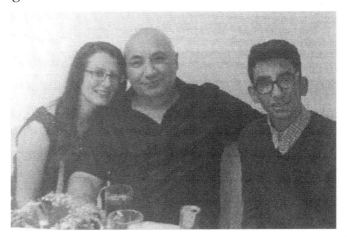

All is well.

CHAPTER TWENTY-THREE

CHILDLESSNESS AND MEN WHO WANTED TO BE DADS

Dr. ROBIN HADLEY[20]

"You are a man because you have children." (Dyer et a, 2004) [21]

In March of 2016, we were in London with Andrew Bridgen[22], MP for North West Leicestershire, a brilliant person who went out of his way to help us launch *AIEWWTBCM*. We had some pictures taken outside the Department of Health that he used to issue a press release.

---

[20] Dr Haley's website http://www.robinhadley.co.uk/

[21] Dyer, S. J., N. Abrahams, N. E. Mokoena, and Z. M. van der Spuy. 2004. "'You are a man because you have children': experiences, reproductive health knowledge and treatment-seeking behaviour among men suffering from couple infertility in South Africa." *Human Reproduction*, 19 (4):960-967. doi: 10.1093/humrep/deh195.

[22] See: http://www.andrewbridgen.com/

There, we had the privilege of meeting Kate Brian, a representative of Infertility Network UK, and the owner of the blog *Fertility Matters*[23]. During the meeting, she asked Mr Bridgen to champion the postcode lottery in relation to IVF. As it stands, depending on one's postcode, you can have more or fewer funded attempts at IVF, which is a very unfair system. Kate became a mom through IVF, and she is still out there, helping people going through this torment. Selfless and dedicated! She was also kind enough to put me in touch with Dr Robin Hadley who has done a study on childless men.

Before I continue, I want to point out something. When we were trying to get pregnant, I was motivated by the desire for my wife to find some peace so that we could move forward. Had we not had children, I would have been upset just because Vas would have been upset. It is as simple as that. I never had that longing to be a father, and the fact that it looked as though we were not going to be parents made it a moot point. However, there is a big difference between imagining something and actually seeing it materialise in front of your eyes. It puts things into perspective. For me, it happened when Vas got pregnant with Xristos. At that moment, I knew that in a few months, I was going to be a father. That was when the longing came. I had always thought that this longing belonged

---

[23] http://fertilitymatters.org.uk/

only to women. Ignorance in its purest form! Yes, I am still learning and appreciating other people's pain.

When Kate first introduced Dr Hadley and me, it was as Steve and Rob. When Dr Hadley got in touch with me, he signed off as Rob. I still did not know who he was. I thanked him and sent him the manuscript. The shop was busy, so it took me a couple of hours to have a closer look at his email. I got his surname and looked him up on the Internet. I read his impressive bio, and to my horror, I read that he'd never had any children. I immediately sent him an email explaining that, even though I was going through the pain of my experience in the book, I did manage to become a father in the end. I did not want to upset him by reminding him of what he wished for and never got. Still, he was strong and gracious enough to read it. A shining example to us all.

This is Dr Hadley's article about childless men:

I Always Expected to Be a Dad.

I am an involuntarily childless man. In my thirties, I was desperate to become a dad, but through a "constellation of circumstances," did not become one. I was born into a large family of eight children in a working-class area of Manchester in 1960. My whole life, I'd expected to be a dad, and my reactions to not becoming one included anger, depression, elation, guilt, isolation, jealousy, relief, sadness, yearning, and withdrawal.

After working as a scientific photographer for thirty years, I left my safe job to study. First, I studied counselling (Hadley, 2008), then research methods (Hadley, 2009), and finally a doctorate (Hadley 2015). I came to study involuntarily childless men through a throwaway comment.

Searching for a topic to research for my counselling degree, I casually said, "I was very broody in my thirties." The tutor looked surprised and replied, "Never heard about that before—do that." That tutor was Dr Liz Ballinger and she set me on a most unexpected journey. I thank her from the bottom of my heart.

It was during that first research project that I found that there was virtually no research into men's desire for fatherhood (Hadley and Hanley, 2011). I also found out that I was not the only man to feel extremely broody about wanting to be a father, not that you would know that from the general media. Nor will you find much about the male desire for fatherhood in academic or medical sources. Most of the work in those fields is concerned with women and motherhood, though the number of studies focusing on fatherhood is increasing. Within the wide range of work concerning infertility, the vast bulk centers on the experiences of women.

Men want to be fathers. Not all—but most. In fact, the level of desire for parenthood in childless men and women who want to reproduce is about the same (Hadley 2009).

It is, therefore, a myth that only women want to become mothers and that men "are not bothered" about becoming fathers. I have interviewed many men about their involuntary childlessness. The term "involuntary childlessness" is usually associated with people who have accessed infertility treatment that was either unsuccessful or that they withdrew from. However, there are many people who wanted to be parents that did not access treatment, and who may see themselves as involuntarily childless. This chapter draws on my interviews with men, some of whom have accessed infertility treatment.

I focused on the following broad questions:

What do men who wanted to be dads but did not become them have to say about fatherhood?

What is their lived experience?

What are their stories?

The men I have interviewed had a wide range of feelings and thoughts about their desire for fatherhood. Jeremy (63) described an almost physical yearning: "I really do need to have these children."

Similarly, Ben (63) noted the hurt and regret: "I felt the pain of it, emotionally there was a real gut feeling that I'm not the father of my own children."

According to Shane (33), fatherhood would provide many benefits: "You need to have a child to make you blossom as a person and as a family."

For Phil (51), being a father would connect with his own experience: "You know I'd look at my son growing up and remember me relating to my dad. My dad was a good dad, enjoyed being a dad. He was delighted to be a dad. And I'd always assumed I'd become a dad."

All the men to whom I spoke assumed they would become dads and that their lives would consist of: "Leaving school, getting a job, finding a girl, getting married, buying a house, and having a family."

These are the words of Martin (70), who had always wanted to be a dad. After marrying for the second time in his forties, he and his wife Mauve tried for a family before accessing IVF treatment. It was at this point he found out he was infertile, and they decided to try donor insemination. Martin admitted that he struggled to come to terms with not being the child's biological father, but Mauve's right "to experience motherhood" was the priority. After a couple of attempts at IVF, they both agreed that the cost of the treatment in terms of stress, anguish, and pain (as well as money) was too much. Martin describes the grieving process he went through: "What it does to you emotionally… it took me a while to get my head around…not having children. What is worse in comparison? I think the secret, in the end, is acceptance. 'Yes, I'm really not going to have children.' You have to get over the denial and go through a process of emotional tempering. Eventually, you come out of the other side." Martin adds, "It is something I will never stop regretting. You know, it won't go away."

There is a common assumption that people who don't have children, at some deep-down level, did not really want them. However, my research shows there are many factors that may influence whether a person has children.

John's story shows how both wider economic and very personal factors affect parenting plans. John (60) and his partner got together in their mid-twenties. They both wanted children.

"I said, 'Well, two would be nice.' She said, 'Four would be better.' Well, I just thought, 'I didn't think life could be this good,' but it didn't worry me."

John and his partner worked hard and bought a four-bedroom house for the children they were going to have. National economics made them delay having children.

"The bloody interest rates went up to 13 percent! We were working all the hours just to keep a roof over our heads! So, we delayed trying for children."

Having survived that financial crisis, John's thoughts turned back to parenthood. Now in his mid-thirties, John is aware of both the biological clock and of the socially acceptable age for being a parent.

"I said to her, 'We just don't want to let time go by and let nature take the decision from us.' And so she said, 'Well, I never thought you are responsible enough to have children.'"

John's experience highlights how circumstances affect people's opinions concerning parenthood at different times during their lives.

The impact of not keeping to the expected "work/partner/accommodation/family" ethic was also apparent in Shane's (33) life. At school, aged ten, Shane was in class when his teacher asked what they wanted to be when they grew up.

"My hand shot up, and I said, 'I want to be a dad!' Everyone started laughing."

At age eighteen, Shane's life plan was to go to university, start a career, get married and, have "two children by the time I was thirty."

He accomplished the first three of those ambitions, but not achieving the last had a very deep effect. Shane's first marriage ended when he was in his late twenties, following the strain of infertility treatment. His second marriage, after repeated miscarriages, ended eighteen months prior to our interview. Shane was very aware of time.

"I am very impatient now to start the life I should have had. I was very, very, depressed, devastated—suicidal last year."

A Swedish study (Weitoft, Burström, et al., 2004) found that lone fathers and childless men have a higher rate of suicide and risky behaviours than other men.

Shane went on to explain that one of the reasons why time was so important was because, "You're young enough to it [fatherhood] before you're too old."

Similarly, Marcus (33) highlighted how the end of a recent relationship had made him realise how much he wanted to be a dad: "When that relationship ended, I felt a huge loss, as I had lost the chance of having a family."

All the men I have met were aware that parenting was not easy—as Marcus said, "The sleepless nights and the nappy changing—that would be hard."

They all noted that there were advantages to not having children. Marcus said, "It's been easier for me when I've changed jobs and move." However, each man has said that they would have preferred to experience fatherhood.

I have been privileged to interview men about their childlessness. Almost all of them had one thing in common. They all said, "This is the first time I've talked about this."

All the names of the men interviewed have been changed. The fluctuations of normal speech—hesitations, the "um"s and "err"s—have been removed for the sake of clarity.

References:

Hadley, R. A. (2008). Involuntarily Childless Men: Issues surrounding the desire for fatherhood. MA Dissertation, The University of Manchester. Hadley, R. A. (2009). Navigating in an Uncharted World: How does the desire for fatherhood affect men? MSc Dissertation, The University of Manchester. Hadley, R. A. (2015). Life without fatherhood: a qualitative study of older involuntarily childless men. PhD, Keele University. Hadley, R. A. and T. S. Hanley (2011). "Involuntarily childless men and the desire for fatherhood." Journal of Reproductive and Infant Psychology. **29**(1): 56-68.Weitoft, G., B. Burström and M. Rosén (2004). "Premature mortality among lone fathers and childless men." Social Science &Medicine. **59**(7): 1449-1459.

Dr Hadley is giving speeches and lectures on this topic. It would be nice if a publishing house decided to publish his extensive research. It will help men going through this pain—they will know they are not alone.

Reading Dr Hadley's story enabled me to see things I had not considered before. I now know that many men go through this pain when faced with a childless future. As I did not have that yearning at the beginning, I hadn't considered the devastation a man can live with when facing a childless future. I cannot imagine my life if I was not a father—it is what defines me. It has brought fulfilment and completeness to my life. My heart goes out to the Hadleys of this world.

I have already mentioned birthday parties and christenings. Another possible source of pain is Father's Day (not forgetting Mother's Day). You buy a card and a present for your dad; you want to celebrate and acknowledge your gratitude to him for bringing you into this world and for all he has done for you. You write that card knowing full well you will never get one. You have regrets, and you think life is unfair, but you never let on. You smile while your inner being shreds. This is the kind of pain that in a twisted way reappears year after year to torment these poor souls for what they wished for and never got.

Another realization engulfing childless men/women is the knowledge that with their death, their bloodline ends. There will be no descendants down the line to become the next

Ghandi, Mandela, or Mother Theresa. Knowing that infertility can take the future away can be soul-destroying.

You can be 'childless-by-choice' and you can be 'childless-by-circumstance.' In the former people take a position that they will *not* become a parent. In the latter, there is a large range of circumstance that means people don't become a parent. That choice is taken away from them.

Childlessness is a loss. It is the loss of the baby you will never have. It is the loss of the future you wanted your life to take. It is the loss of a part of you. It is the loss of hope, dreams, and laughter.

In my opinion, like any loss, you should cry, get depressed and mourn. You will be submerged in futility, helplessness, and nothingness. There will be mornings when you will not be able to get out of bed. You will be thinking, "What is the fucking point?"

Before you attempt to move forward, deal with this mourning. You will hit rock bottom, and you will be overcome with anger, hate, and injustice.

Accept that:

*you will never get the chance to love, guide, and nurture the baby you will never have.

*you will never hear the laughter of the baby you wanted, echoing around the house.

*you will never read him/her a bedtime story.

*you will never take him/her to school.

*you will not give him/her away at his/her wedding.

*you will never have your grandchildren stay overnight.

*you have nothing to be ashamed of.

*you have been robbed of the noblest of dreams.

*sometimes life just sucks!

*you will have a split personality. One that projects to everyone that you are okay and the real one that suffers from a broken heart.

You might be thinking that what I am saying is easier said than done. I know it is hard, but you don't just owe this to yourself but also to your wife. If you feel crashed for being childless, imagine how much worse she is feeling. Deal with this loss for your sake as well as hers.

 Once you accept it, then and only then, you may have a chance of somehow rebuilding your life.

Know this: in the years to come, you will learn to live with pain. It will never go away but instead it will linger around like a noose ready to tighten and stop you from breathing, when an idiot like me asks you if you have kids (see Epilogue). You will tell him 'no' and put a fake smile on your face, when all the while your first instinct is to grab him by the throat.

I have read an article in the Guardian by Stephanie Marsh in which Dr Hadley Hadley gave his point of view regarding 'The desire to have a child never goes away'[24]. It was heartbreaking.

Dr Robin Hadley: this gentle man; this giant, is dedicated to his cause to inform people of the pain of a childless future.

I shall now compare two people's approaches to infertility. One of them will shine, while the other falls to pieces.

Dr Hadley wanted to be a dad and unfortunately did not succeed. He learned to live with it. He got on with living a productive life by becoming a doctor of social gerontology, maintaining a happy marriage, and still positively touching other people's lives. He never lost himself, even though his main regret in life is not having a child. This selfless man gives lectures and speeches about childless men, helping other men to deal with this kind of profound loss.

Assume I did not manage to become a father. It would have meant the end of my wife. By now, you know quite well who and how I was. You can bet your last penny that I would not have done nearly so well as Dr Hadley had I failed to have a child. I would have sold everything, disappeared, and would

---

[24]https://amp.theguardian.com/lifeandstyle/2017/oct/02/the-desire-to-have-a-child-never-goes-away-how-the-involuntarily-childless-are-forming-a-new-movement

have only brought misery and destruction to the lives I subsequently touched.

Dr Hadley helps and educates; for me, there would have still been that group of people I intended to visit and then transcend to become the lowest of the low, for I am dedicated. All this would have taken place because of the wrong steps I took at the beginning that changed me. Do you see the difference between Dr Hadley and myself? There was no excuse. This change in my person was down to me and my self-importance. *I was the king!*

This is why meeting people like Dr Hadley gives me hope. I feel privileged when such people take the time to talk to me.

CHAPTER TWENTY-FOUR

<u>I AM MY FATHER'S SON</u>

"He lived his life on his own terms."

This is an extra chapter which I had no intention to share; but for death. So here I am telling you about my father. It is Friday the 27th of October 2017. Sadly, he passed away four days ago.

From the young age of eleven, he had to drop out of school and be the breadwinner of his family. He missed out on so much in his life and I think it had a huge effect on him. He was a man of a few words, inflexible in his views and with a very short fuse. He was giving, never intruded into anyone's life and he was also funny in his own unique way. To his dying day, he lived his life according to his own values and with very few regrets. His world was black or white. There was no gray. He either liked you or he ignored you. There were no half measures. He was a tough man; a man's man. He never shouted; he only had to glare at us and we toed the line. Up to the age of fourteen I wanted to be like him.

Even though we knew he loved us, he had never said it. He never hugged us. I understood why. He never experienced it as a kid and didn't know how to deal with it. He was also not one for mushy stuff. When I was twelve he enrolled me in a private school. He came from humble beginnings but he wanted the best for us. Through sheer hard work and determination, he formed a company which to this day is very successful.

We had a lot of arguments, during my teen years; I was a rebel. I wanted to debate things and my father tolerated no discussion; his word was law! He didn't know how to express himself. I wanted to buy a motor bike. He said 'no'. No debate. I wasn't okay with that. The following week I got a weekend job as a waiter at a café. When he finished work, I told him that I needed a motor bike to get to work as that would've enabled me to be around tourists and practice on my English. He agreed and he bought me that bike. At the end of the second shift I quit that job. He knew I had manipulated him but I would like to think he liked my fighting spirit.

I thought I was different from my dad. I was articulate and I knew how to express my views.

On Monday, I was supposed to drive Vas to hospital in Birmingham. Instead, late Sunday afternoon I was tearing down the M1 and M25 trying to catch a flight to Cyprus from Gatwick airport, leaving for the very first time Vas and Petros by themselves.

Seeing him lying in that hospital bed, with that damned monitor bleeping like crazy; that the heart it was monitoring, was not beating any more filled my eyes with tears. The last two times I cried was eighteen years ago, when I begged the doctor not to give up on my son and when I drove Andrea back to our local hospital. Including this one, these are the only three times I cried in my life. The last time I heard bleeping monitors was when Petros was born. Hearing my dad's monitor bleeping, paralysed me. It brought back so many bad memories. It felt as if the sky was falling on me, crashing the life out of me. I could not breathe. I felt all panicky and the feeling of doom was overwhelming. I just had to talk to Petros and make sure that he and Vas were okay. Phew! He answered his phone on the first ring. They were still driving to Birmingham. I asked him to give me a call every hour until they arrived safely at home.

That Monday morning I cried for my father whom I have never kissed on the cheek. I cried for the opportunities lost and the realization that I can never rectify it. The mixture of emotions was overwhelming. Of course, me being me, I never cried in front of my family. When I couldn't take it anymore, I would pretend to look at my mobile as if I was going to make a call so as to leave the hospital room and then the tears would pour uncontrollably. I was a mess. I've learned to share my emotions in front of Vas and Petros but that's about it.

Looking at my dad, I realized something; the reason we clashed was not because we were different. It was because we were the same. My world is also black or white.

"I am my father's son" and I am proud of it. Just like my dad, regrettably, I have never told him that I loved him. I never hugged him. The only physical contact we had was a hearty handshake. Apart from Vas and Petros, I've never allowed anyone to hug or kiss me. Man or woman, I always stretch my hand for a handshake.

Petros idolized my dad. When we were in Cyprus on holiday, Petros would sit next to my dad for hours, listening to his stories. Of course I was there to interpret. Whenever he ran out of stories, I told him to make one up. He would glare at me and tell me, "You know quite well, I don't make stories up. Do you want me to tell lies to my grandson?"

All I could hear was Petros telling my dad, "More, more stories granddad."

"Well, if you don't want to lie, you better remember one sharply, because Petros has given me a headache."

He would smile and instantly the new story would start. Apparently he wanted to create suspense. For a person who had never spoken more than ten words in one go, give him a beer, his grandson and he would talk for hours, about things that happened in his life which I had never heard before. It was as exciting for Petros as it was for me.

I explained to Vas and Petros why I am the same as my dad.

Vas chuckled, "I have been telling you this for years. When you are angry you press your lips together just like your dad. Your stubborn streak is just like your dad. You are not very talkative with strangers."

I smiled, and not wanting Vas to continue, I looked at Petros, "The smartest thing I have ever done in my life was marrying your mom. Had I married anyone else, I would have gone through life unable to express my feelings."

Vas was not ready to let her statement halt, "Your eyes that piercing look when you are furious, just like your dad."

"Yes, but when I am around you two, I am at my best!"

Vas smiled and nodded.

I always tell them I love them and the hugs are in abundance. I always explain to Petros why I said 'no' to something he asked for, and we debate it until I am sure he understands my point of view.

Petros has grown in a loving environment and I am sure he will be a great dad when he has his own kids.

I married his mom, who insisted on sharing my feelings and communication. I adapted and the things that my dad did which I did not like, I tried never to repeat. What's more, as Petros is like me, I told him that the things I do that get on his nerves, to remember them and never to do them with his kids. He has to do better than me.

My dad had the excuse of a tough upbringing. What was my excuse? I conveniently found excuses to avoid telling him those four words. It felt as if it was not very manly telling him, 'I love you dad'. Plus, it also helped when I thought to myself, "I'll tell him next year on our next holiday. It's not the end of the world."

Guess what! The years went by and I said and did nothing. He is now dead. There is no more next year. Time has caught up with me now. There is only guilt and fucking regrets. Seeing him lying there and knowing there is no more tomorrow but only the memories of all the missed opportunities filled me with shame.

I am my father's son:

*I am sorry for the things I said and especially for the ones I didn't say.

*I am sorry for the things I did and especially for the ones I didn't do.

*Yes, I love you and I am sorry you have not heard these words from me while you were alive.

God Bless you and may you rest in peace.

CHAPTER TWENTY-FIVE

<u>MY PERSONAL OPINION</u>

"We are all born special."

I believe that every single human being is special. We all come into this world pure of any prejudice and hate. You just have to look at babies and the abundance of love they give. They give it without reservation or conditions. Everyone is accepted and loved by them irrespective of their color, size, religion, and sex. We are then exposed to prejudices from possibly our very own homes, friends, schools, workplaces, and experiences. When we allow them to influence us and take our "special" away—it is our choice and ours alone.

What stops us from being special are the actions we take in our daily lives that have a negative impact on others. Whether you sell drugs, steal, kill, lie, bully, be dismissive, racist, or feel superior to others, it is your choice. The actions you take show your character. You can try to excuse your behaviour by saying you didn't have any other choice or by blaming it on your upbringing. These are all excuses to justify your weak nature and poor choices in life. Other people in similar circumstances have chosen a different path. I can definitely tell you that I was not special. . Don't be like me. It is not too late. Be a good human being.

You get on with life by taking steps towards your goal, whatever that may be.

Every step you take will affect the next one. You will find that taking the wrong step is quite easy. Often, taking a positive step requires hard work and putting yourself out there. Seeing a homeless person and stopping to give him/her some money is more difficult than just walking past him/her.

The step you take today that will influence the step tomorrow depends solely on you. What do you want from life? Do you want to leave your mark on this world? Or, on the other hand, do you want to go through life as if you never existed?

The other day, I saw a documentary on the telly about a guy in London who is schizophrenic. He was on the London Bridge, planning on jumping to his death. Many people walked past without even a glance. They either never saw him, or if they did, they pretended they had not. Finally, one man stopped. He spoke to the schizophrenic man for a long time until he persuaded him not to give up and not to make that jump. The documentary covered the schizophrenic man's efforts to find that stranger. They did meet, and it was emotional to see them talk about what had happened.

When I heard that guy say, "I thought to myself, I am not letting you die today, mate," it sent shivers down my spine. He did not pretend not to see him; instead, he touched the life of that stranger. Should that person have kids or positively touch other lives, it will be because of the selfless action of that man who stopped that day, preventing him from killing himself.

However, the steps I am talking about here are about having a positive impact on your family and not strangers. Easy choice, is it not?

For some people, it will be difficult to get pregnant, and others might face what Vas and I faced. You have my sympathy and understanding. I hope none of you make the mistakes I made.

When you try to create life, the most sensible thing, in my opinion, is to be prepared for the worst. I am not a pessimist, but a realist. If the worst happens, you accept it and deal with it in a strong frame of mind, thus enabling you to be a better husband to your wife, for she deserves nothing less.

The first thing you need to understand is her need to be a mother is not an unreasonable obsession, but rather a part of who she is. By appreciating first the depth of that desire, you will become more understanding of her depression and frustration. By reading about possible difficulties, you empower yourself.

Don't believe me? Google search "infertility/IVF destroyed my life," and you will see the heartbreaking stories of people who split up due to infertility. These are only a small fraction of the real number. Countless other couples split up for this reason without anyone knowing.

The bottom line is; why did you marry her? Was it only for the good times? This period is probably the only time your wife will truly need you, for she is a tortured soul.

Remember, you said, "For better or worse, in sickness and in health." Never take the first wrong step. Never be as I was.

If you are working for a company, you will put in the long hours to get that promotion or an increase in salary. You can be away for days because of a trip your boss requires you to take. If you are willing to do this for your job, what extra lengths are you prepared to go for your family?

Whatever you learn is never wasted. If you try to have a child but cannot, the lessons you've learned will hopefully help you never to take the first wrong step. If you never face any of these problems, your kids and grandkids might. Be there for them, and share your wisdom, thus preventing them from taking the first wrong step as well. I can include friends and family. Always tell them, "Don't be like Steve."

We keep hammering that we are the protectors of our family. Governments have the army to protect the country and the police to protect their citizens. What safeguards have you set up to protect your family? How are you going to minimise difficulty and avoid divorce? You can bury your head in the sand, hoping that you will sail through it. I think that is wrong. I did exactly that, and you saw where that got me. Be the protector, and not just in words! You take this first positive step, making it more likely for you to take another one. I took the first wrong one, and it snowballed from there. The decision is yours.

Some men (especially me) find it hard to show and to share their feelings. Look at me now. You could say I've verbal diarrhoea. We are no longer living in the dark ages. You are not weak, though some may think you are. Do you really care? Your wife will not think that, and she is the only person whose opinion counts. Your family comes first, second, third, and always.

Most of us at one time in our lives have lived through a horrible experience. Some will seek therapy, while most will just continue without dealing with what happened. The baggage of that experience will hang over them, possibly for the rest of their lives. If you are like me, you might not want to tell a complete stranger your most private thoughts. If you still want to deal with it, put it down on paper. I don't mean try to get it published; write it for yourself. Pour your heart out, but write down the exact feelings you had at the time, irrespective of whether they were good or bad. You might feel it is a waste of time, or you might find it daunting. Persevere. I hope you find it as therapeutic as I have. You will be able to deal with your demons and will hopefully feel an invisible weight lift off your shoulders.

I can hear you telling me, "Steve, I have lived through it. I have not forgotten. Why waste my time putting it on paper?"

The forgotten things you will drag up once you start writing will amaze you. Just put down what you remember, irrespective of whether it is in sequence or not. Keep writing new things and, at the same time, go back every now and then and try to expand on what you have already written. Put it away somewhere for a time and forget all about it. Then try reading it again as if for the first time. You will be amazed. I was!

Live through your pain again. Digest the whole period, and try to figure out if you made any mistakes. Accept them for what they are without admonishing yourself, and learn from them. Try not to repeat them again. This is what I am doing.

Learn from your mistakes so that in a few years, you don't find yourself sitting in a dark room all by yourself, trembling, crushed, and trying to figure out where it all went wrong. It went wrong because you took the first wrong step. Whether that was cheating, lying, hiding your true feelings … well, the choice was yours.

I told you that my greatest shame was lying. I have accepted it, learned to live with it, and vowed to never repeat it.

Reliving the past, I came to realize something very disturbing. It is something that never once crossed my mind during those years and, until today, I would have found it absurd even to consider it. Well, today is the day of reckoning.

Vas needed protecting from me.

She needed protection from the man who claimed to love her, protect her, and be there for her, no matter what.

How is this for self-analysis? To actually come to the realization that, for all the bullshit of presenting myself as Vas's protector, I was a failure in that as well. When you brush things under the carpet and avoid dealing with them, you never gain any self-knowledge. It is only when you face the past that you realise how time can make you forget what really happened. It is only when you face yourself that you finally see that you've had a distorted and biased view of your own past. *I was the king!*

Take the first right step today. Don't put it off until tomorrow, or you will find another excuse not to start.

You can try and ignore your pain as it is no longer there

or better yet, pretend it has never happened. You can suppress it for a while. I think you will be fooling yourself if you think it has gone. It lingers around like an invisible noose. I got on with life, going to work every day, enjoying and loving my family. I honestly thought I was unaffected. However, there was always a heavy weight on my shoulders. There were always dark menacing clouds hovering over me. In complete denial, I dismissed them. I always prided myself on my strong mind and steel style character. Time has a funny way of always catching up with all of us.

There were two choices. Continue the same path as before oe deal with my baggage. I stood my ground and faced my past and my shame. I think it's the only way to help one's self. Lay it all out, accept your shortcomings and mistakes. Learn from them with the hope it will make you a better person, husband and father. Your family deserves nothing less.

I'll tell you about a couple who are regular customers at the Moira Chippy. The woman has read *AIEWWTBCM* and told me how happy she was that we'd shared our private story. They're a very nice couple and have two young boys. On the outside, you would not think a tragedy had befallen them. This happy-go-lucky mother was once on the receiving end of an accident caused by a careless driver. She was in a coma for some time. When she eventually opened her eyes, she did not know who she was. It was months before her memories returned.

As if that was not enough, she had to learn how to talk and walk again. It was an uphill struggle, but she persevered. Her husband decided to write a book about it. It has been three years since he started. Looking after the boys is quite demanding, and he feels there are not enough hours in the day to accomplish this task.

Whether he finishes it now or later, it does not matter. He keeps writing things down as and when he has some free time. It may take him a few more years to finish, but the important thing is he has taken the step to deal with the painful times he had to live through. He is dealing with it, and he might help other families facing this type of tragedy. He has reportedly found it quite therapeutic.

The effect it had on me was quite unsettling and rewarding at the same time.

Since writing these two books, I remembered things I thought I'd forgotten forever and things I'd consciously tried to forget. I was happy dealing with the forgotten memories, and on edge dealing with the intentionally suppressed ones. In the end, I dealt with both sorts with a rare kind of passion. I relived the past with the hope that it would help shape the future. Ours is a very personal story, and I could have quite easily left it for my eyes only. The thing that made me decide to publish was simple: as I was reading it, I felt it would have made our journey easier if I had read of someone else's real-life experience. The hope is, these books might help even one couple from making the mistakes I made.

What you will read below may sound old fashioned and outdated. First, live for a few years with your wife and go through some tough times. If you have kids, it is because she gave birth to them and most probably she is the one who made adjustments in her working life, (going part-time or giving up work altogether). If you never managed to have a baby, you will see the daily pain that she has to live with. Whichever path your life takes, you will not be able to help yourself. It is in your genes. You will want to be her protector and rightly so! It is not because you think she needs protecting. It is because you feel you have to.

For the Female Readers:

I believe that most married men want to be their wives' protectors. When circumstances prevent a man from doing exactly that, he will see himself as a failure. When he sees you hurting, he hurts too. First, because he sees you suffering, and second because there is not a damned thing he can do to help. If he is scared, he will never admit it, for he will wrongly think it will portray him as someone you can no longer lean on. Men as creatures may be stubborn, but they are definitely not complicated.

You might be facing a terrible situation, be it infertility, bankruptcy, or conflict. Your husband might not be very forthcoming in giving his point of view; his responses to your questions might be grunts. He might even pretend he has not heard you. It will most probably irritate the hell out of you, but don't despair.

It does not mean he does not care or he is not listening. He is probably scared and hurting inside, but he does not know how to open up. He wants you to always know that you can lean on him. Wrongly, he might see emotional eloquence as a weakness. Behind the confident and uncaring persona lies a worried and scared man. He needs help but does not know how to ask for it. He will move heaven and earth for you. He stupidly expects you to be a mind-reader.

Men are from Mars and women are from Venus. It is up to you both to gently break those stupid barriers.

The only time he is not listening or looking is when you ask him if your shoes or handbag go with the dress you are wearing. Vas is forever asking me this. At one time, Petros was standing next to me.

"Dad," he said, "you haven't even looked! Why did you say yes?"

Busted! "Your mom has been asking me this question forever. Back in the day, the couple of times I stupidly voiced my opinion, we were late leaving the house because she had to change her outfit. In the end, after changing a few times, she still wore the same dress and told me I did not have a clue. Whatever she wears, I am okay with it as long as she is ready on time. It is easier to just say yes."

Petros laughed, and Vas threw me a dirty look.

But men do care when you are hurting. Sometimes our pride and inability to show our emotions will make us come across as uncaring or indifferent. This is not true.

Yes, on this one, please, help us. Don't give up on us.

IMPORTANT! *Don't wait until you have a problem and immediately expect him to open up. It will not happen. Start today! Share your feelings and emotions about silly and serious things. Ask him to do the same. He may be reluctant at the beginning, but try to break down those barriers. Men are creatures of habit. Once he gets used to this kind of environment, it will be the norm for him. You deserve nothing less.*

Try this: Ask him to read this book and then invite him to give you his thoughts. If he is truthful, he will say, I was weak for letting the process overwhelm me but in agreement for withholding the truth from my wife. Tell him this, "I heard that Steve is quite stubborn, scary, unyielding in his views and tough [it is true]. He was not overwhelmed because of what happened. It was because of the wrong steps he took. Simple things like sharing his feelings and emotions with his wife and lying. I don't ever want you to be like Steve."

You have read what problems I have lived through. Granted, I created some of them through my own stupidity. Depending on how easy or hard your journey is, your husband will at least face a mild version of my struggles. He might be as terror-stricken as I was.

During the "puppet times," if you see a change in his facial expression, even for a split second, tell him, "It's okay. We can do it tomorrow. Let us have a break tonight." By trying to understand how he feels, I am sure he will reciprocate.

You will be enduring the pain of infertility, IVF, pregnancy, and actually giving birth. You will shine in your selfless attempt to be a mother and a creator of miracles. He will be shining as well, but his inability to show his emotions will be blocking the light. He will see your pain and torment, and it will tear him up inside. He will want to take it away, for seeing you hurting is torture for him. Seeing him looking strong and unaffected is the filter that prevents you from realizing how much he cares. He is suffering as well.

As a matter of principle, I have never bought my wife flowers on Valentine's Day, nor have I taken her out for a meal (apart from the first two years when we first got together). Someone telling me when to buy my wife overpriced flowers or take her out for a meal is not something I can get on board with. I say this to my customers, and they are surprised she is still with me. Actually, I am surprised as well! What I never tell them is that I buy her flowers every week without fail because I want to and not because I am supposed to.

I don't finish work until quite late in the evening. When in bed, Vas might sometimes ask me for a cup of tea. I smile and get up to do it. She is my wife. Period. At the shop, it is a different story. I tell the customers that I may sometimes wake her up at three o'clock in the morning and grunt, "Tea." In my fabricated story, Vas obediently gets up and gets it without protest. One guy was quite impressed but luckily, his wife, Tracy, was with him. In a no-nonsense manner, she told him that if he ever does something like that, she will kick him out of the house

Tracy, "You can go and live with Steve if you dare pull that macho crap on me," she told him as she glared at me.

One of the girls jumped in to spoil my fun: "Don't believe Steve. He is kidding. He will do anything for his wife. He buys her flowers every week and still tells people on Valentine's Day that he does not buy her any."

Tracy bought *AIEWWTBCM*. She asked me to sign it, telling me with a grin on her face that, "If you die, it will be a worth a few bob." I was not impressed.

After she read it, she asked me why I told her husband the story with the tea.

Smiling, I told her, "It was just a joke—anyone who actually behaves like that does not deserve his wife. Anyone who is influenced by someone else's macho crap is weak. Anyway, Andy is not like that, and you know it." Whenever she is at the shop and hears me tell that story, she rolls her eyes and smiles. I'll have to fabricate another story soon because everybody has heard this one.

The new one I recently started is, "In my next life, I want to come back as a woman!" The reaction I get from the women is amazing.

First, they roll their eyes. They then give me a look as if they were talking to a complete idiot. They are not sure whether to pity me or slap me.

"Why would you want to do that?"

"Mainly because odds are, I'd have a full head of hair, headaches ..." Their main response is, "You will be disappointed," followed by an angry look. The ones who have read the first book know my views on women and the suffering they go through. They just sigh and say, "Here he goes again!" If there is a new customer, as soon as she jumps up to argue with me, the other women put her straight, saying I am teasing. I feel lucky I was born a man and would not in a million years want to come back as a woman. I can hardly cope with my "man flu", never mind having to deal with periods, hormones, trying to get pregnant, pregnancy, giving birth, and menopause. Women are made stern stuff.

For the male readers:

When I first started in business, I planned to own and operate multiple outlets. It's difficult to achieve this, but I knew I could do it. Work hard for ten to fifteen years, own a portfolio of properties, and then take it easy. You keep knocking on the door of opportunity so you can achieve your dream. I was young, and the world was my oyster.

Battling infertility obliterated all my business plans. How could I think of expansion when my wife was depressed? How could I attempt to work longer hours than I was already doing when my wife needed me to be there for her? Facing such a battle changed my priorities. Things I considered important before became irrelevant. The door I have been knocking on became a brick wall, and it no longer held the allure it had at the beginning. I actually took a 180 degree turn away from it, as my goals were no longer on that road.

As you know, life held no meaning for me back then. Business was a necessary task I had to perform in order to pay the bills and buy food. That was it. This kind of change in attitude was forced on me by the new course my life was going. I had two businesses and a house. I would have given them all up in a heartbeat, if that had enabled me to see a smile on my wife's face by having a baby.

By the time Petros was seven years old, we were confident he was progressing steadily and that we had weathered the storm. I was tempted to resume my dream of expansion. I had a chat with Vas who only said the following words, "Life is what you make it. What do you want from life?" She did not object to my plans, but she never directly answered my question either.

We were riding the good times now, and I forgot that I was willing to give up everything so we could have a baby. We now had Petros, and here was me wanting to work longer hours, getting more stressed, and in effect be away from my precious family.

I smiled at her and said, "You are right. We are okay as we are."

Wise beyond her years. I can still tell the time with my moderately priced watch, and I can still drive from A to B with my average car. It's not the amount of money you have that matters; it is the quality of life you are giving your family with your presence and unquestioning love. The end result was me spending more time with my family. You can't compare money with happiness. You can't let the years go by thinking you have time to make amends for the times you were not there for them. Once you miss it, that is it. Whether you are the richest or poorest person in the cemetery, when you are dead, you are dead.

The moral behind this is, how have you utilized your time when you were alive? Have you always been there for your family? Have you loved them with all your heart and have you been loved back? If the answer is 'yes', you are rich beyond your wildest dreams, and you don't need money to make you realize it.

I have a friend, Vic Waghorn[25], who is an actor. He shared something the other day which I think is spot on. I am going to summarise it here:

"Imagine that there is a bank that credits your account daily with £86,400. You cannot carry forward to the next day any unused amount. Use it or lose it. You would make sure you draw out all of it, wouldn't you? Each of us has such a bank. Its name is time. Every morning it credits you with 86,400 seconds. If you don't use it wisely, it is your loss and yours alone. Invest it to get the most out of wellness, happiness, and success. The clock is running. Make the most of today."

As you know, I felt I neither needed nor did I give support to anyone. If you were to have met me back then, you

---

[25] See http://www.vicwaghorn.co.uk/

would have thought that I was just a deranged person. You would have formed this opinion by just looking at me as I would never have allowed a conversation to start; I would have hated you. That was just me. *I was the king!*

Other men going through this journey might fittingly need moral and spiritual support. Why? I have already talked about infertility (puppet times, firing blanks, angry and depressed wife and pressure from work). Add to this the experience of IVF.

They might also be affected by something unthinkable and unexpected . Their mental health. It was true in my case. My mental health (and my wife's) took a bashing of epic proportions. Anger, hate, shame, loss of faith, and tilting to insanity. I never thought it would happen to me, but it did. We all think we are tough and strong, but we all have our breaking point.

I have mentioned couples splitting up because of infertility/ IVF. It is a tough situation to be in, and couples need all the support they can get in order not to become part of the divorce statistics.

There are infertility/IVF support groups for women, and rightly so. However, there is hardly any support for men. Men's suffering goes almost unnoticed. They might keep quiet about it, but they are suffering as well. They need support to help them get through this experience. I am sure I would have dealt with my situation better had I been a member of such a group.

You cannot very well tell your friends that your wife is pushing you to the edge with her depression and mood swings. You cannot tell them that you dread going home as you are feeling like a puppet when she is ovulating (I was the king!). You just can't. They will not understand that you are just venting your frustration and will most probably think you are heading for the divorce courts.

Men need support from other men who are in the same boat as them. Total strangers, who will not pass judgment, and who are going through the same things with their own wives. They will know it's not just them going through this experience. They will find out that it's not just their wives who are depressed and angry. Knowing and sharing these things will empower them with extra strength to fight the good fight and really be there for their wives.

However illogical it was, my wife held on to that fertility doll. Was it wrong? Of course not. It gave her comfort and hope. As long as they were positive feelings, she could have had twenty of those dolls as far as I was concerned. How about me? Once we went to see Professor Nicolaides, I saw him as our good luck charm. It was illogical but it gave me comfort and hope as well.

My story has somehow had a positive outcome. It might cause pain to someone still struggling with infertility and IVF. I do hope that it gives them comfort and hope. If we somehow managed to survive our journey, I sure hope you survive yours as well. I wish you success in your journey.

The following is very important not to mention. When I first met Vas, she was working as a bank clerk. A few yearsmafter we got married she decided to stop working, and I was okay with that. By default, I became the sole bread winner and I thought I was the one who was working hard. *I was the king!*

It was and still is as if I am living in a five star hotel with a concierge. My thinking at the time was that as she wasn't working, she had a lot of free time. I was sure I wasn't putting her out, if I wanted a meal (kleftiko) that took five hours to prepare. *I was the king!*

Look around you. The house is clean and running like clockwork. Your kids are fed and happy. Do you know how much work it takes to achieve this? When Petros was five years old, Vas fell ill and had to stay in hospital overnight. I had to look after Petros. Petros wanted cheesy pasta but as I have never cooked, we went to a restaurant. At home, after watching cartoons he went to bed. I think I had about two hours sleep that night. Every half an hour I would go into his room to check that he was okay. I was shattered. Vas, like every other woman, does this every day. The house doesn't clean itself. The meal doesn't appear on the table out of thin air. Your baby will not turn into a teenager all by himself/herself. You will only notice that things are not done when she is too ill to do them. What about if she isn't a housewife and she is working as well? Your wife is your partner in life. Like every partnership you have to do your share of the work.

Once you walk in your house leave your anger and stress from work outside. Kick to the curb your macho crap. Turn your mobile off. Don't go out with the guys for a few drinks. If you want to go out, go with your family. Do you know what kind of door is, the front door you have just entered? ? It is the front door to 'Heaven'. Embrace and cherish what you find in your house. Give them your undying love and constant attention. You are lucky; because for all your shortcomings and weaknesses they are still there and they still love you (it is true in my case!)

If you are at work and you cannot wait to finish and go home to be with your family, in my opinion, you have cracked the simplest and most important part of married life.

EPILOGUE

"Vas is the beacon to a better me."

A few people have told me that they would have enjoyed this book more if they had heard from Vas. I agree! Vas only spoke about our experience in AIEWWTBCM and has no intention of doing so again.

I have written this book for one reason; I hope it will help other people avoid making the same mistakes I did. On a subconscious level, I think I have also written it for my wife. I wanted to tell her that I know and appreciate what she has done for us. I've tried to say this to her a few times, but my words failed to express my gratitude and my regret for failing her, correctly. Every time I start, she laughingly tells me, "Don't go soft on me Ferengi. Your race is ruthless." I have done here exactly what my mouth failed to put into words, but the sad thing is, she will never find out.

Know this; whilst you have almost finished reading this book, my wife will not have read the first page. She will never read this book as it relates to our painful past. It breaks my heart knowing this. I wanted her to see me for who I really was and not who she thought I was. Evil is the word to describe me. She is a gentle soul who suffered greatly. She sees the best in people. She actually sees the best in me. I am grateful for this, as she does not see my weaknesses and shortcomings. Do I have regrets? You bet! Have I failed her? You bet! For all my mistakes, I have done one thing right in my life. I married wisely.

Before you even contemplate trying to get pregnant, make sure you get the fundamentals right.

Marry wisely: The most important decision you will make in your life is the woman you choose to marry/partner. It is not what job you take, what house you buy, or what hairstyle you choose. Don't rush into it. You are not getting a car knowing that in a few years you can trade it in for a newer model. This is for life.

Forget the fairytale romance you see in films or read in books—such relationships don't exist. If you do decide to marry for just looks, you are in for a shock. You will find that time will not be kind to either of you. Choose unwisely, and you will face a miserable married life or a quick visit to the divorce courts.

Pick the woman who makes your heart skip a beat. Don't look at her body, hair, size, color, or wealth. Close your eyes, and let your heart make the decision. Don't confuse lust with love. Find your soul mate. Be thankful when you wake up in the morning and you see her still lying next to you. She has agreed to spend the rest of her life with you. Appreciate her, and don't take her for granted. Life can be tough. Facing your trials with the right woman by your side will empower you with immense energy, determination, tolerance, understanding, compassion, and love. I never experienced much of these things until I got married. Vas is the beacon to a better me. Make her your queen and the center of your universe, for she deserves nothing less.

Before I got married, I had an idea of what kind of a husband I was going to be. Let's call this model "Husband A." I was certain that the woman I eventually married would not be disappointed. I was that husband for the first few years with Vas. Unfortunately, infertility intruded into our lives and changed me. Enduring those eighteen months of IVF and birth made me worse. I was a disgrace of a husband and became "Husband B."Writing this book, digesting that period, and reliving the pain, torture, and her flirtation with death obliterated Husband A. That man is no more. Contrary to what I thought at the beginning, he is not good enough to stand by Vas's side anymore. I changed after realizing I was not worthy of her. Every day starts with me thinking, *what special thing can I do for her today?* Granted, most days, everyday life gets in the way, but I am still trying to be a better husband, for she deserves nothing less. My wife, like your wife, graced us by being willing to spend the rest of their lives with us. It is a privilege and an honor, and we should act accordingly. Relive the past, remember their selfless actions, and feel lucky that they accepted us into their lives.

Share everything with your wife: You need to tell her all your insecurities and fears. She is not a mind-reader. She also needs to know precisely what is happening. Don't use the excuse, "I did not tell you because I was trying to protect you." There is just one word for that: "Bullshit." She is not the little woman in the house whose only function is to keep the household running and be available in the bedroom. She is your partner in life. Treat her like one. As my father-in-law says, "Two heads are better than one."

Love thy neighbour: If you live through an intense situation, accept and give support to others. Bad things happen to everybody, and they need your support as much as you need theirs. The world does not revolve around you.

Dealing with our situation was tough for me, and I am sure it would have been the same for any other man. My mistake was amplifying the problems through my wrong steps. You have already read what I think I should have done. Every action you take has a consequence. Had I started with the first right step, I would not have found it so overwhelming. Wrong steps pushed me over the edge, causing me to become an antisocial monster. You can say it was self-inflicted, and I would agree with you. The instigator was my stupidity, selfishness, ignorance, and self-importance. Yes, I suffered like most men would, but I have no sympathy for myself. Am I in the minority? I hope so! *I was the king!*

I wish Xristos and Andrea were alive and with us. It was not to be. I miss them terribly. It would have made Petros's life easier, having his brother and sister around. Instead, he is our only surviving child and, unfortunately for him, all our attention is on him twenty-four hours a day. Sometimes I get on his nerves with my suffocating attitude, but he knows I am scarred.

Petros is eighteen years old now. I have always talked to him in an adult manner, even when he was a kid. Eleven months ago, the two of us went to town, as Vas was not feeling well. While I was driving, he told me something that shocked and saddened me. It still amazes me how kids think it is their fault when their parents divorce or something else bad happens in their family.

"Dad," Petros said, "for as long I can remember, Mom has had health issues."

"Yes, I know."

"Is it because she got pregnant with me?"

"You know what happened, right?"

Petros nodded.

"It is a lot of things. It was a long struggle for her. The constant frights she faced, the IVF chemicals, and the trauma when she thought you'd died after we brought you home shook her to the core."

"I am sorry," he said.

"Why?"

"For being the cause of her ill health."

"I am surprised you said that," I said. "I have told you the story enough times for you to know that you have nothing to be sorry about."

"Yes, but it all started with me."

"It started way before you, mate. Your mom had about ten years living on a rollercoaster of shitty things happening. She lost two babies. She was willing to die for you. Do you think that just for one second she's had any regrets?"

"I cannot help feeling that if it were not for me, she would have her health."

"You are so wrong. If it were not for you, she would be dead. Try to understand this. If you had not survived, the happy atmosphere you see in our house today never would have existed. You gave her hope and, because of you, we are where we are today."

"Why does she not talk about it then?"

"You know that she still has nightmares about it,

right?"

Petros nodded.

"It affected her badly, and she cannot talk about it. Doing so will force her to relive those times."

"How come you were not affected by the whole thing?"

I laughed. "I am damaged goods as well, but it was not me who did the hard work. It was all your mom."

Petros was quiet.

"Instead of you saying sorry, here is me telling you 'thank you' for keeping us together. Never think it was your fault. You are wrong! Your mom was willing to die for you. Having a few health problems is, I guess, a small price to pay."

With time, I hope he comes to realize how precious he is to us. Whenever I introduce him to anyone, it is with pride and a smile on my face. You would think I'd taken all the risks and done all the hard work!

This is how selfless women are.

Love, honesty, compassion, sharing, communication, and commitment are the least they deserve.

I have a healthy fear of dogs. Big or small, they sense my discomfort and growl as I approach, which scares me even more, thus resulting in more growling and barking. Getting a dog was something I was always against. After a few years of badgering, Vas and Petros wore me down, and we got Brian (named after the dog in Family Guy). I guess whatever they want, if I can afford it, and it is legal, they can have.

Vas is besotted with elephants. Thank God it is not legal to have one in the house! Instead, I commissioned a painting by our local artist, Cristina, depicting VASPX as a herd of elephants. Vas was in tears when she saw it. It was quite a surprise! It is just one tiny attempt to make it up to her for what she went through for us.

We have a private joke. Vas sometimes calls me an alien. She finds the fact that I never shout unsettling. She might be screaming at me, but always I respond in a quiet monotone, which infuriates her even more. She will continually ask me why I don't shout at her when I am angry, and I tell her again and again that I do enough shouting at the shop, especially when suppliers increase their prices without informing me. She will always ask me why I don't do it with her.

My answer to her has been, and always will be, the same: "Because you are my wife!"

I always say that to her with a smile on my face. Some days she will come over to kiss me. On other days, she will call me weird. In the end, however, she always settles on "alien." She claims I am a Ferengi, after my favourite character Quark from the *Star Trek* series, *Deep Space Nine*.

Up to this day, Vas has never realized two simple things

about me. I am not a complicated character. What she also failed to realize was that I was, and still am, happy. Why? I got the girl!

Two years ago, when we were visiting my in-laws, I tripped and fell on the concrete floor outside my brother-in-law's house. I was holding my cigar in my left hand, so without thinking, I tried to break my fall using only my right hand so as not to damage the cigar. Yep, pretty stupid. My wrist swelled. When I finally got to my in-laws, I was in a lot of pain. Vas offered to go to the chemist with my mother-in-law. I just crashed on the settee feeling sorry for myself.

Five minutes later, my mother-in-law runs in the house shouting, "Steve … Steve … come quickly, Vas had an accident with your car."

I jumped from the settee and started running out of the living room with my wrist hurting like crazy.

I asked her, "Is Vas okay?"

She said, "Yes, she is alright. Your car is not, though." She was panicking, as she always did when under pressure.

I immediately stopped running and started walking. It was more bearable as my wrist was throbbing.

She shouted at me, "Why are you walking?"

"As Vas is okay, there is no need to run."

Eventually, I arrived and saw that the passenger side was

mercilessly scratched. Vas had decided to get quite friendly with the wall on their drive. She looked a bit unsettled. I smiled at her and told her not to worry. I managed to get the car out of the drive and drove with her to the chemist. My mother-in-law was surprised—she'd expected me to be angry.

In the car, I was laughing. "Once your mom told me you were okay, I started walking, and she got upset with me."

"She was worried you were going to get angry with me about the car."

"As long as you are alright, why would I get upset about metal?"

"God, you really are an alien," Vas said. "But you are my alien!"

Xristos and Andrea died. I'd almost lost Vas and Petros. Cars, money, and houses can be acquired again and again. Vas can call me an alien all she likes, as long as when I go to bed, she is lying next to me, and she is the first person I see when I open my eyes. I consider myself the luckiest and wealthiest person in the world. I wish you the same!

Whether we like it or not, life follows a cycle of highs and lows. It happens to everyone, not just to you and me. You may see a celebrity wearing a Patek Philippe watch and driving a Lamborghini. Jealousy might be the first thing you feel, but you don't know what risks they took or what sacrifices they made to get where they are. Irrespective of their fame and wealth, their lives follow the same cycle as yours. Instead of drowning in jealousy, do something constructive to change your own life.

In the morning when you first open your eyes, thank God for giving you another day to enjoy. When you turn around and see your wife lying next to you, smile, give her a kiss and tell her "Thank you" before you even wish her good morning. You can still tell the time with your moderately priced watch. With your average car, you can still get to where you need to go. Love your life for what it is. You are alive, and I hope you have married wisely. Feel lucky and realise as well as appreciate what you have. It is priceless. Make compromises and sacrifices (make it work for both of you!), and show her she has married wisely. Don't leave it until tomorrow. Now is the time!

If you are single, and you woke up this morning with no one special lying next to you, put this book down and go and find your girl. There is a time to be single and play the field, and there is a time to find that special someone. Get to work. Now is the time!

I married wisely. Did Vas? That is a question for her to answer. Through Vas, I became a father. Petros, my beacon, is here with us and doing quite well. Xristos and Andrea are our angels. I achieved all this through Vas. If I got the girl, why would I ever raise my voice at her? If my girl is sad, how can I not automatically be sad too?

After reading about our lives, you might romanticise a false picture and think our marriage is great. You are wrong! It is like yours. We have our arguments and fallouts too. After every argument, we clear the air and move on. What we have learnt from our life experiences is that life is fragile. We embrace and cherish what we have with a passion.

When the time comes, my wish is that Petros will marry wisely as well.

Another thing I would be remiss not to mention are the couples who tried to achieve their dreams of having a baby and never succeeded. God bless you, and I hope you find happiness and fulfilment in other avenues. Some decide that adoption or surrogacy is the way for them. Others try to cope with the emptiness. You tolerate it because there is not a damn thing you can do. Does the pain get any better with time? Maybe, but it only needs a trigger for all the emotions to come back.

A few years back, we were at a friend's wedding. I was talking with someone who kept referring to teenagers. It was quite loud there, and I don't hear well at the best of times. I thought he was talking about his kids, and I naturally asked him how many he had. To my horror, his facial expression changed for a split-second. I knew I had made a big, insensitive mistake. They could not have kids. He told me it was okay. He made a joke of it, but I knew I had probably spoiled the evening for him. I was thankful that his wife was not with us at the time. If he were anything like me, he would have given me a spine-chilling glare for upsetting her. He was a teacher, which is why he was referring to kids. It was my stupid mistake. I apologised and, to this day, I have never asked anyone about having kids without being 100 percent sure beforehand. Even if I see kids with them, I wait until they refer to them as their own.

We had a terrible time, as many people do, but we brought Petros home in the end. That couple had been through the wars as well, but they have nothing to show for it. It is not over for them. There will always be an idiot like me who will accidentally bring to the surface their pain. Many years go past, and this heartbreaking and gut- wrenching desire never leaves them. Over the years, they attend christenings and birthday parties. Never be one of those people who spoils their evening by reminding them what they failed to have. Never forget this. Be special. My heart goes out to them.

You have the whole picture now.

The funny thing is, my wife was the one carrying the weight of our family all by herself, and here I am writing a book about how I suffered. However, irrespective of the depression, pain, and brush with death that my wife went through, in my own way, I suffered as well. I was not the confident and self-assured person that I intentionally projected to her. I was petrified. Most men going through this kind of journey will face a similar ordeal.

You might still face problems further down the line, but both of you are strong. You will not let this problem defeat you or break you up. God forbid, you may never get to achieve your dream, but your strength will keep you together as a couple. You can explore other paths that might fill the emptiness.

When you go through this process, whether it is painful or you sail through it, you face this journey as a strong, loving, and compassionate unit. It is no longer a question of who is suffering more. Your unit as a whole is suffering, and together you remain strong and unyielding.

I wish you success and happiness on your journey. I hope you sail through yours without any complications and stay true to one another.

I made many mistakes with Vas. Yet, whatever mistakes I made, my heart was in the right place.

The last statement I want to make is this: Vas and Petros rock! Xristos and Andrea are our angels. I got the girl, and I am a dad!

We suffered. We fought to achieve our miracle. We are VASPX.

This is my family:

My wife's name is: **V**aso

My daughter's name is: **A**ndrea

My name is: **S**teve

My son's name is: **P**etros

My son's name is: **X**ristos

We are   **VASPX**

God Bless you all.

I hope you have enjoyed the book.

It would be great if you could take the time to leave a review for *I Only Wanted to be a Dad*. Every review matters.

If you did not like it, please, say so in your review.

Should you like it, and you feel it might help others, please, leave a review, mention it on your social media platforms, and tell your friends. Unknown to you, you might get to help someone who is going through this struggle. **Yes, be special!**

You can also visit www.vaspx.com and sign up to our newsletter. You will receive updates of upcoming books and more posts on marrying wisely.

I think this will be the next book: **I Only Wanted to Marry Wisely.**

More books by VASPX:

1. *All I Ever Wanted Was to be Called Mom*

2. *Realms and The Curse*

3. *Realms and The Giant's Spear*

Steve has had his fill of real life, pain, and scares. You can now join him and his group of fighters battling King Maxwell in order to stop him from becoming immortal and taking over the world forever. You can read all this in the *Realms*, a young-adult fantasy series.

You can also find him on:

LinkedIn: Steve Petrou

Twitter : @vaspx

27243085R00172

Printed in Poland
by Amazon Fulfillment
Poland Sp. z o.o., Wrocław